A GUIDE FOR EQUINE SOFT TISSUE REHABILITATION

The Plan Book

Rebecca Kells Brotemarkle

author·HOUSE®

AuthorHouse™
1663 Liberty Drive, Suite 200
Bloomington, IN 47403
www.authorhouse.com
Phone: 1-800-839-8640

First published by AuthorHouse 1/13/2009

ISBN: 978-1-4389-2811-1 (sc)

Printed in the United States of America
Bloomington, Indiana

This book is printed on acid-free paper.

Library of Congress Control Number: 2008910147

DEDICATION

I realize, at this stage of my life experiences, that "dedication" is without a doubt the most important word one will have to understand to be successful at any aspect of life. Dedication is understood best by the circumstances for which someone chooses to involve him- or herself.

Check the dictionary and you will find among the definitions of *dedication*, a commitment to a particular course of thought or action. I feel this definition is the truest for this book, and I feel complete in the understanding of this definition. It is also an invaluable and important word for my readers to appreciate and embrace.

As far as to whom I dedicate this book, without hesitation, I must start with my veterinarian, Dr. John Lockamy. He embodies the definition of dedication. He may not realize the level of knowledge he has given to me, nor does he live by the rules, but he finds the exceptions and thinks "outside the equine box." John Lockamy is by far the most dedicated, passionate, and committed veterinarian I have ever had the pleasure of knowing. His sensitive commitment to veterinary medicine is unsurpassable. He is kind and always has vast amounts of information to share with his equine colleagues; you learn to understand the total equine if John is your veterinarian. Those who are willing to learn appreciate the insight John will give them; those who do not will appreciate his veterinary talents for their horses' needs.

What I am telling folks is that those of you who do not want a formal education in equine management may not understand the wacky world of equines and the people who are involved with the evolution of the sport, and those who are an integral part of the entire functional matrix of this sport. We need a bit of every type of people in this crazy business; it keeps us working, happy, and above all helping and understanding the horse—our athletic partner—and his needs during an injury. So, first I must give Dr. John Lockamy his just dues. He has exceptional, dedicated family values, and sacrifices many a family hour to stay with a client on a Sunday night colic case.

Next, I must be very thankful to my wonderful husband, Eric. His patience and kind understanding are rare; he has a true gift of real love. Most men are very confused, annoyed, or frustrated with the horse hobby of their significant other, and it can become a huge source of conflict for many couples. Not my sweet Eric. He is beyond wonderful; he had gotten frustrated many times with the entire rehabilitation process, but he never complained, and that is the most important thing. This time and therapy I spent with my horses simply just needed to be dealt with, and he accepted that. Eric was such a silent strength for me, without even knowing what that meant to me at that time. He was less interested in the success of the business; he loves the horses and he loves me. That is all that matters.

I know I am a very fortunate woman.

Next, I must dedicate a few words to my friends Sarah and Arlene, for the many long-distance phone calls and tears of frustration that they shared with me. They never had to understand the level of frustration I was going through; they only had to listen and say, "I know, Becky; I know how hard it is." Sarah herself has been laid up because of various injuries, so on many levels, she could identify with my situation. Arlene is a phenomenal physical therapist for human patients; she hopes to bring the merger of veterinary medicine and equine PT into a much-needed awareness. She too is an amazing, dedicated, driven, and devoted equestrian whom I have the pleasure of knowing. She has given me such insight and depth of knowledge of the functional changes that occur during this time. She has introduced into my world the understanding of structure and function of the horse.

Thanks to Miss Kit at Lady Jean Ranch for being so patient for my loss of clarity, and in knowing the oddities, beliefs, and demands that my horse and I needed at this time. She is the most fantastic farm manager any facility could have. She was a level-headed voice and a friend. She does not realize the magnitude of her being, but those of us at Lady Jean Ranch do; that is why we are there. She is the common thread linking everyone at our particular facility together, and should be an ambassador for her negotiation skills and diplomatic prowess as a performance horse farm manager.

I also have to mention my farrier, who understood the level of hoof management that needed to be dealt with. He never let me give up. Bob Corey knew this and managed my horse commendably during a very long and difficult time. He has been with me for ten years, and I have dragged his butt everywhere up and down the East Coast. Thanks to his gifted talent, he helped me manage Buddy through this time. Bob did this because he believed in me and Buddy, not because I could afford the luxury of a personal farrier. He knew it was not within my means, and I must thank him for his devotion to the horse and give him respect for the fact that he is not a dinosaur, but a timeless antique.

A word to my parents: I know to this day you have no idea about what this entire book is about, or my equine fascination, but perhaps being the defiant child that I am, the rebellion became a driving force in my education. I must thank you for being my parents, and I must thank you, for giving me the opportunity for my equine passion to exist. I was supported by the position you provided for me. I had the resources to have horses, and I must let you know *how grateful I am*. I appreciate the opportunity to make this book and my equine obsession evolve, and I thank you so very much for that.

I need to mention Dr. Robert Scott of Fort Lauderdale, a gifted veterinarian and equine chiropractor. Along with the progressive massage talents of John Pierre Hourdebaigt, the author of *Equine Massage Awareness* and the guide to a well-informed complete body program for equines and humans too, these two gentlemen have become my most recent guides to the equine healing arts available in the ever-so-evolving relationship of equine rehabilitation and supportive friends.

I must lastly thank Dr. Gregory Fowler of Ocala, Florida. He has been a great influence in my education of equine rehabilitation management as well. He was supportive, knowledgeable, and holistic in his approach to veterinary medicine.

I was very fortunate to have many who deserve this dedication, and I know the friendships I have are special. Dedication is the first word of my book, and is truly the word that makes this time successful. These are the people who have taught me to make my dedication a reality, and hopefully a guide for others to utilize when they are rehabilitating their own horses.

From the words of Francois Robichon de la Gueriniere: "Horsemanship is the one art for which it seems one needs only practice. However, practice without true principles is nothing other than routine, the fruit of which is strained and unsure execution, a false diamond which dazzles semi-precious connoisseurs often more impressed by the accomplishments of the horse than the merit of the horsemanship."

Table of Contents

Introduction
It All Began With A Horse

I am writing this manual with the hope that my ideas will encourage and guide amateur horse owners and trainers of all disciplines toward a successful recovery from soft-tissue leg injuries for their equine partners. It has been my experience that there are limited **real-life** resources available to help us plan for the unknown future of amateur rehabilitation. The resources I found were very insightful as to the healing process, medical/anatomical references, and success rates. But there is very limited professional information offered and very little attention about the daily management, care, "physical therapies," and reconditioning exercises. Most of the information I found available was focused on the racehorse industry. Granted, they may be the *largest* discipline for observing soft-tissue leg injuries, but other disciplines experience the same soft-tissue leg incidents as well. The injuries and rehabilitation program I am addressing involve individual owners, with far less experience than the professionals of the racehorse industry. Most horse owners have very limited experience in any form of medicinal equine management, never mind the entire soft tissue rehabilitation process. Our veterinarians during this lay-up time will visit us about every thirty days and comment on the healing process and check the progress of the injury. But most doctors do not understand, are not experienced with, and are not trained to comment on the daily challenges, and appreciate the nursing and management of what will become "our" daily circumstances, emotions, and potential *life-threatening safety issues* from dealing with this scenario of equine rest and rehabilitation.

This is a significant statement and must be acknowledged during this process.

If you and your horse live at a boarding facility, your "barn friends" (others who share the barn) may seem to have some possible insights for you, but unless they have experienced this situation, their skills are limited.

The trainer and manager of your barn may see you obsessively walking and hand-grazing your horse, two to three times a day. You will become focused and disciplined and not be able to have idle chitchat when you are handling your horse. You may need to explain to them that you must have your attention completely on your horse during this time.

If you have your horses at your home, someone you know may be able to give you some more advanced handling tips. Your horseless friends will question your reasoning as to how much time this will demand of your life.

It is my hope to share with all types of horse people my insight and experiences, to give veterinarians a layman's resource of daily soft tissue management and provide some know-how for those people who need the information.

You must truly understand—this is not an easy task or any one person to do, an experienced horseman or a casual owner.

Understanding what you have to manage and what you have to deal with on a daily basis, with the possible career-ending situation you are in and dangerous challenges mean:

- You *must* educate yourself in all areas of rehabilitation.
- You may have never wanted to know as much as you will learn about the horse's limbs. But you will need this information.
- You *must* have control of the horse's power and the mental state your partner may take.

- You *must* use the proper handling equipment, the proper drugs or other types of medications and above all make the **safest** decisions.
- Your horse deserves that you learn all these areas of rehabilitation; only then can you truly help him. Unless the injury was caused by an obvious accident or poor conformation challenges, some external factor caused this. Take responsibility for your partner. Do not throw him in the field; this is not vacation time, especially for the sport horse.

Every horse-and-owner combination is unique,
and every rehabilitation situation is different.

All of life's factors will be of great importance during this process. The climate, season, and environment, and the personality of you and your horse will decide and affect your program. Above all, the amount of involvement **you dedicate** to your horse will make this time the greatest success. Every day, you will need to re-assess this lay-up time; you will alter and re-evaluate your program as to the best decisions for you and your horse. You will develop a program of ideas that work best for you. You will also have an array of armchair experts who think they know what is best. But the bottom line comes down to this: Have they been in your shoes, and what was their success rate? Only that person with true advance experience may have an idea or two that you could use. This manual is a reference to help prepare you for issues that may arise. I didn't develop this plan; it developed itself. Through the daily rehabilitation process and my learning to survive the unexpected day-to-day, the ideas became reality and lent themselves to this guide. Because there will always be another horse lover, rider, trainer, owner who will find him- or herself in this situation.

Unfortunately, the everyday routine will become very lonely and very much about you and your relationship with your horse.

You will feel ready to give up a million times and lose clarity.
This is a trying time and an unpredictable
one as well.

Safety is above all the most important factor—safe handling, awareness of conditions, and the healing environment. This guide does not guarantee any miracles or fast healing.

EVERY FACTOR NEEDS TO BE DISCUSSED WITH YOUR VETERINARIAN. THIS BOOK IS NOT A SUBSTITUTE FOR PROFESSIONAL MEDICAL ADVICE.

This book is merely an account of my experiences.

Even in the best of circumstances, there is the possibility that you could get hurt or killed and your horse could become dangerously unmanageable. This is a bold statement, but I believe it is necessary for my readers to understand.

This manual does not guarantee that my ideas are the best. I would be a fool to make that statement in a book for the horse industry. But it is my hope that I can provide each person who will go through any soft-tissue leg injury rehabilitation a reference and realization that he or she is not alone. This *can* be done, and your time, decisions, and attention will make a difference as to the success of your horse's recovery.

During this rest and rehabilitation time, it will be **imperative** that you find resources and professional healers. I have such great admiration for the team of professionals who have helped increase my equine education. You must be able to feel you can ask many questions of these professionals; do not take at face value that every "professional" is educated in how to properly manage a soft-tissue injury. Ask your veterinarian to help guide you with this area of education of your horse's situation. Your veterinarian should help you understand how and why there is no such thing as "quick fixes" in this scenario. The methods you choose to utilize and assist the healing process will be significant, but remember the most important and the best remedy for this situation is patience and the tincture of time.

You may now find yourself at a time when you need to ask your friends and family for patience. If you are a trainer and your show horse is presented with a situation of rest and rehabilitation, your equestrian clients will have to accept even more obsessive equine-related behaviors than they did before. I have been beyond frustration at numerous times, and then had to hear the random comments from folks who were sharing their "helpful" remarks. This was not healthy or positive in a time that requires support and not criticism. "Retire him," they would say; "He is a cripple"; "He is too old"; "He will never be able to be competitive again"; "Turn him out, and leave him alone, then bring him back next year." I disagreed completely with all of these comments, and some days, these comments were very difficult to deal with during this year of healing.

But in the larger picture, a year passes too quickly.

All of this I heard, and the comments usually came on the worst days of the rehabilitation. I had been angry and in total disbelief at how my veterinarian expected me to actually accomplish this overwhelming task.

Not only was I angry, I was without any help or experience in this area of equine management—and I am **a certified USDF dressage TRAINER, a certified equine massage therapist, and have interned as a veterinary technician! I have a BS in animal science, with a veterinary concentration. But this was a situation of horsemanship that was completely foreign to me.**

As I have learned, no person realizes the seriousness and depth of this time as much as you, the injured horse's owner. No one appreciates how **your** horse awareness skills become elevated to the most extreme levels. The ignorance other people have as to how dangerous a situation you are in every time you take your horse out of the stall will be eye-opening. They won't understand why you will go ballistic when some other horse owner just wants to let his horse get some bucks out and lunge, while you are walking your laid-up horse. Nor will anyone understand how crazy you become when the owner of the facility decides to refurbish the landscape and have dump trucks of dirt delivered when you are just starting to trot your horse that has been in his stall for twenty-three hours every day for the past six months. This becomes a very sensitive time mentally, physically, and emotionally.

Much hope and support do I have in my heart for you, my equine friends, and my readers for a safe recovery. It is my goal to offer you support and comfort in this very, very long and frustrating process. Some of the readers' horses will be very good patients, and you will breeze (sort of) through this time. Exceptions exist, but most horses do not read the book on perfect equine behavior. Breed, temperament, and environment are very important factors; your capabilities as a horseperson are as well.

So read on, and apply some of my thirty years of horsemanship, and multiple successful soft-tissue injury recoveries, as a guide that will offer you a direction for a healthy, safe, and sound recovery.

Rehabilitation is a lonely time, and I want you to consider me an empathetic friend during this time. You will get to know some of the dirty little secrets of horsemanship and realize someone else, somewhere in this horse world, has gone through this time too.

Be honest with yourself during this time as well. You may not be the best person for this job. Do not be afraid to send the horse to a rehabilitation clinic if this task is too overwhelming.

**_Recognize: You are not a failure for
realizing your limitations._**

CHAPTER ONE
Let Us Begin: Education

DEFINITIONS:
TENDONS CONNECT MUSCLE TO BONE;
LIGAMENTS CONNECT BONE TO BONE

The "soft-tissue" injuries I will be referring to are known by a variety of names. High or low suspensory, bowed tendon, check ligament, deep or digital flexor tendon, and inflammation of the tendon sheath are the common names. Strain, tendonitis, and tenosynovitis are the formal names. This, in very basic terms, means: acute and/or chronic inflammation of a tendon, ligament, and/or the sheath that the tendon slides in and is in unison with.

The primary role of the tendon is to transmit muscle activity to bone, which will move the joint when the muscle contracts. Some tendons attach to more than one bone, and move more than one joint. Basically, the horse's leg should be viewed as a system of pulleys and levers. Keep this in mind to help understand the locomotion system of the horse.

"Ligaments play a more passive role. Whereas tendons run from muscle to bone, ligaments run from bone to bone, over at least one joint. The primary role of a ligament is to provide structural support for a joint" (*FN Equine Lameness* pages 395-438 Chapter 11 Tendon and Ligament Injuries).

STRUCTURES OF THE LIMB AND THEIR FUNCTIONS

The tendons in the leg can be divided into two types: flexors and extensors. There are two major flexor tendons—superficial digital flexor tendon (SDFT) and the deep digital flexor tendon (DDFT). There is one major extensor tendon—the common digital extensor tendon. These tendons attach to muscles in the upper leg, just above the knee or hock. They then run down the leg and attach onto the pastern or pedal bone. (See illustration on next page.)

In the foreleg, the flexor tendons flex (bend) the knee and fetlock, pastern and coffin joint. The extensor tendon extends (straightens) these joints. In the hind limb, the flexor tendons flex the fetlock, pastern, and coffin joint, but they extend the hock. The extensor tendon does the opposite: It extends the fetlock, pastern, and coffin joint but flexes the hock. When looking at the cannon from the side, the order of structure from front to back is:

* Extensor tendon is attached to the extensor muscle of the fore or hind limb; it is the main tendon responsible for the horse's leg to extend and reach forward. This is opposite when the horse moves his hind limb and his hock; the extensor tendon is contracted.
* Cannon bone is the large bone that starts from the knee or hock and ends at the fetlock joint. Surrounding the cannon bone are the splint bones; they are vestigial bones, which were the toes of the horse millions of years ago. (Prehistoric horses had five toes.) The splint bones—there are two—attach to the cannon bones and "splint" the cannon bone, meaning they are attached to the inside and outside of the cannon bones. They are connected to the cannon bones by the interosseous ligament. This ligament must be noted as a potential soft-tissue injury if the horse "pops a splint." A splint-bone injury must be treated aggressively, as it has potential to become a soft-tissue injury if not treated properly.
* Suspensory ligament connects from the point of insertion behind the cannon and some of the smaller bones of the knee or hock continue down the cannon bone and form a "sling" as a

means of support for the fetlock joint. This ligament wraps around the fetlock joint and pastern bone and is integrated in some of the tissue of the extensor ligament.

* The check ligaments are known as the accessory ligaments; they prevent the entire flexor mechanism from getting overstretched. The superior check ligament attaches to the radius (forearm) around the point where the flexor muscle and tendon meet. The inferior check ligament "attaches at the back of the knee and attaches to the DDFT about halfway down the cannon."

* Deep digital flexor tendons' point of origin is behind the cannon bone, and continues down the leg, the back of the pastern, and then under the navicular bone and ending underneath the pedal bone.

* Superficial digital flexor tendon is shaped like an upside-down Y; it starts at the back of the cannon bone, like the DDFT, and then splits around the base of the fetlock joint, attaching to the pastern bones. The DDFT is wrapped by the SDFT.

Keep in mind this is a three-dimensional object; these definitions are merely to assist in my readers' understanding of the relationships of the structures in the limb.

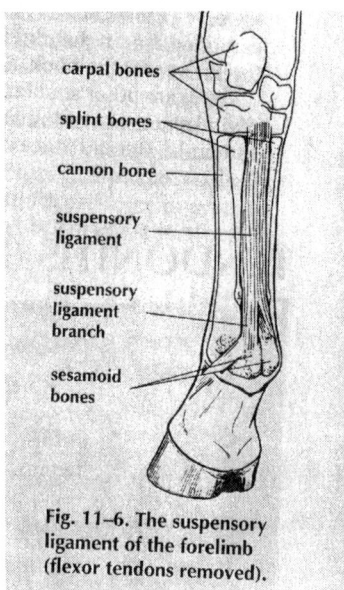

carpal bones

splint bones

cannon bone

suspensory ligament

suspensory ligament branch

sesamoid bones

Fig. 11–6. The suspensory ligament of the forelimb (flexor tendons removed).

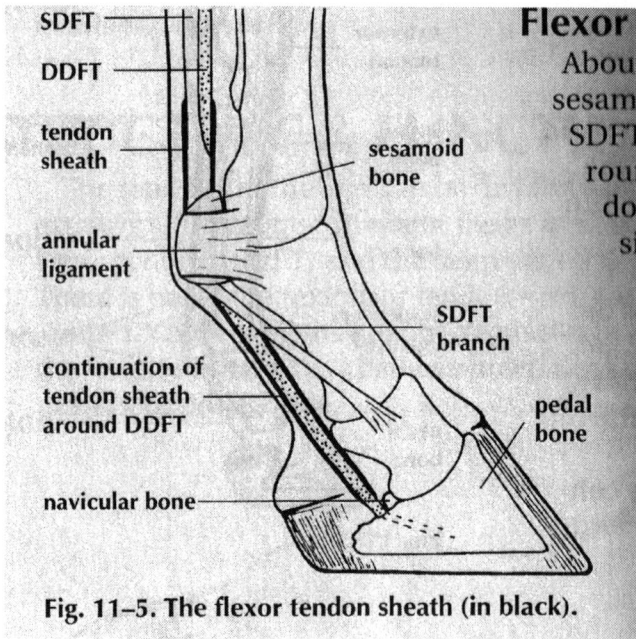

Fig. 11–5. The flexor tendon sheath (in black).

The flexor tendon sheath is in black.

*Notice how the DDFT attaches to the pedal or coffin bone.

(Figure 11-5 and 11-6)
The suspensory ligament
Of the forelimb (flexor tendons removed)

Also make a note of the lack of protective tissue surrounding the limbs. There is hair, skin, and then the tendons and ligaments; there is no fat, no large muscle mass or protection of any sort. This is one of the frustrating aspects of the system of locomotion for the equine; to have a protective surface would prevent the horse from having the ability to move as he does. On the other hand it can be the horse's demise if injured, the proverbial "Achilles' heel."

In my research, I found a book called *Equine Lameness*, published by Equine Research, Inc. Contact Jeanne Wilcox; she is the president of Equine Research. It is a fantastic book, easy

to read, and educates one to the multiple areas of equine lameness. I highly recommend this book for any equine enthusiast.

INFLAMMATION

What is inflammation and what does it mean to my horse and the injury?

Cited from: *General Veterinary Pathology* by R.G Thompson, Chapter 4, pages 152 and 155. Inflammation and Repair states that:

Inflammation is how the body deals with a type of invasion, whether it is from an injury, a chemical, a virus, or a bacterium. This is the body's way of dealing with and repairing the injured area. This includes and involves the vascular and cellular responses in the horse. The purpose of the inflammatory process is to minimize the effect of an irritant to the particular injured tissue. Injury may result in passive and chemical changes in the injured cells or tissues that call forth the inflammatory reaction. The process is recognized as redness, heat, swelling, and pain.

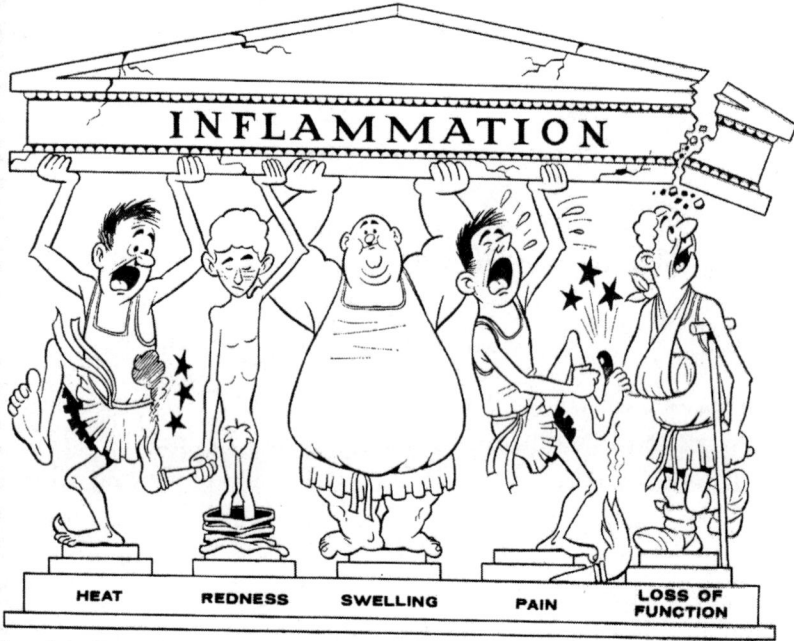

Figure 4–1. The cardinal signs of inflammation. (From Forscher, B.K. (ed.): Chemical Biology of Inflammation. New York, Pergamon Press, 1968.)

He continues to describe that, "The main response to injury is the accumulation of fluids and cells in the injured area. The overall plan for these fluids are to dilute, localize destroy and remove the irritant and to induce replacement of any injured tissue. The fluids and cells together are referred to as exudates, which mean that they have entered the tissue from the blood in an active process. The immune system and the haemostatic functions of the body are often closely involved in the process and this leads to the complexity of interactions."

That is why a complete program with nutritional and physical support must evolve to make your rehabilitation time successful. It is not a time to cut back, but a time to increase your attention to all the systems of the horse.

Types of Injuries

Soft-tissue injuries are categorized by the terminology known as a "grade."

A grade-one lameness or injury is the mildest, and is usually barely detectable by an untrained eye; grade two is still a mild lameness, and usually goes unnoticed by most. If the lameness is categorized as a three, we start to get into a more serious lameness, with very obvious changes in the horse's gait. We may see the head bob—in the case of a front-leg injury, and a hip that hikes higher on a hind-leg injury. A grade four will present usually with the horse not wanting to move or very reluctant to move; finally, a grade five is the most severe and will also be seen as a non-weight-bearing injury. With this type of injury, one will see that the horse will have great difficulty standing up or carrying his weight to any degree.

The most extreme of these soft-tissue injuries is an actual laceration injury from trauma or a rupture injury; any injury that severs or literally explodes the tendons and ligaments will require the most extensive professional medical attention. These injuries require an extremely lengthy healing time, and usually necessitate a surgical procedure. Most of these high-impact injuries are more commonly seen in the racehorse, polo horse, and/or from trauma. These types of injuries can be career ending or limit the usefulness of the horse. The next most severe of these would be any injury that has detached the ligaments or tendons away from the point of attachments to the bone and muscle; sometimes a surgical procedure is a necessary option here as well. Cost factors always need to be considered, and comfortable usefulness of the horse after any severe injury must be a concern. These forms of injuries are best handled by trained professionals and rehabilitators. These injuries are typically referred to as a grade five.

The next type of injury would be the injuries that have holes or tears in the tendon or ligament tissue. How large the hole or tear is and the horse's ability to heal with a supportive program will determine the amount of time off of work your horse will require. Usually, one may remember, see, or feel when this injury happens. These can range from a grade one to a grade four.

The last type I believe is the trickiest to diagnose until it becomes the obvious injury. This injury has occurred very subtly over a period of time. We need to look at all chains of causality for this "not-quite-right feeling."

We must address multiple issues here: our saddle fit, shoeing changes, teeth; does the horse need his teeth floated? Age is extremely important because there are so many changes that occur in the young horse. Did the horse fall down at any point in time? Has our training program changed, or are we facing behavioral issues that were never there before? Keeping all these thoughts in our process of elimination may help us determine there is a soft-tissue injury before it becomes an obvious problem. Other issues arise in our mind during this time of doubt; could it be ulcers or does the horse need his hocks injected again? This is why a mild soft-tissue injury is extremely confusing to diagnose; there are multiple factors that need to be ruled out, and advanced education is necessary to make areas of confusion make sense for the inexperienced horseman.

Horses are very honest about their pain; they do not fake illness or an injury. We sometimes get stuck thinking in our human terms that our horse is being difficult or not doing "want we want." But we must ask ourselves again, are they? Is this a legitimate disobedience or is there something wrong? During this investigation, if a similar factor keeps reoccurring, then it is necessary to investigate that factor. Is it time to realize that these issues may be of larger consequence? Is it a foot problem, a bruise, corn, or abscess? All of these questions mentioned above need to be ruled out as you attempt to determine the source of pain. It can be that old "Which came first, the chicken or the egg?" mystery. Ulcers, behavior, and a "not-quite-right" feeling can sometimes be that soft-tissue injury, antagonizing the horse's surface response in many different ways other than the obvious.

You may or may not have noticed a little heat and a little puffiness in a limb. But a "just-not-right" feeling keeps haunting you. The scariest part of that type of injury is that you usually can ride the horse out of the lameness for a while, sometimes even for weeks! Unfortunately, this has only made the conditions much, much worse. Usually the damage could be minor if we had determined this immediately; now the tendon or ligament has become weakened or even scarred. This creates a perfect opportunity to become a hole, tear, or chronic tissue inflammation.

The reason this initially occurs is because inflammation or fluid gets into the cell walls and expands the structure of the cell wall. Tendons and ligaments are very porous. This fluid weakens the structure of the cell walls, and by not reducing the inflammation from the area, it eventually weakens the tissue, and that is how that little hole or tear is introduced.

This is one of the reasons why some people poultice their horses' legs after a weekend horse show and cold hose the horses' legs after their workouts. Just in case there was added stress on the ligaments and tendons, this cooling practice helps provides relief from inflammation getting any foothold. It is also a good practice to incorporate into any athlete's program. Statistically, we see most of these injuries occurring in the front legs of horses. But this doesn't mean they are not common on the hind legs. It is one of the basic laws of physics: Mass (your horse) plus momentum (his energy) equals an amazing amount of force. Remember watching how fast a horse runs around his paddock and does bouncing stops onto his forehand in the corners of the paddock, as you watch, horrified that he may crash into the fence. Oh, and some horses do crash, so it is a valid fear. That was the basic physics example for the day—mass and momentum in action. This, of course, does not mean every horse that runs the Preakness in his paddock will hurt himself, but it sure could happen. Any slip-and-fall incident must be regarded as a potential soft-tissue injury as well.

Some soft-tissue injuries are from preventable causes: poor shoeing, overweight, deep or slippery conditions, uneven surfaces, overexertion, poor training techniques, and repetitious work programs without overall cross training. Other causes stem from poor conformation and trauma.

Momentum = Mass x Velocity

Chapter Two
Diagnosis

Many mild to moderate soft-tissue leg injuries are often treated too casually, even as far as getting the veterinarian to observe the horse in a lameness evaluation. The rider explains to the veterinarian that the horse is "not quite right." Nothing obvious is apparent, just a "feeling" the rider has. **Listen to yourself.** Now, recognize that not all these feelings are soft-tissue injuries, but this is a factor that needs to be crossed off the laundry list of possibilities. This "observation" cannot be made without palpations or a plan. Some veterinarians casually fall into a two-week **"wait and see"** mode. This resting time may be the correct answer for many individual and casual horse owners, but I have found **MUCH** fault with this prognosis for performance horses. A lack of follow-up and an owner/agent who is uninvolved in the daily monitoring of the two-week "wait and see" procedure can be a recipe for disaster.

There must not be a casual approach to the protocol of rehabilitating a suspicion of a soft-tissue injury.

I am a very firm advocate of taking a proactive approach to any soft-tissue injury defined as suspensory, check ligament, deep flexor, digital flexor tendon, or tendonitis. Whether it is the sheath of the tendon or the tendon itself, these are to be treated very con-

servatively and yet very aggressively. In my knowledge, these injuries become chronic or a long-term problem because they are not handled properly from the onset of diagnosis.

If your veterinarian has diagnosed your horse with any of the aforementioned injuries, you must understand that a **month** of down time will be needed at the **minimum.** You cannot underestimate the seriousness of the injuries without the experience.

Do this time off for yourself and your horse. You may be able to walk under tack, but there must be no resumption of serious work for a month. Two weeks' rest, two weeks' rehabilitation. Resumption of work should only be granted following a veterinarian's approval and an acceptable ultrasound. This method of diagnosis is the best.

FORMS OF DIAGNOSIS:
LAMENESS EVALUATION:

This exam should include an evaluation of the horse's walk and trot gaits; sometimes this will involve the canter gait. These should be performed in a straight line using a halter, lead line, and a handler who provides absolute control of the horse. Some exams may be performed without a rider; some veterinarians may require the horse to be examined in his working tack. Some veterinarians may like to see the horse work on the lunge line as well. The use of the lunge is the best for viewing canter work. The horse will also present lameness differently on the limbs in different directions.

FLEXION TEST:

This testing of both front and/or hind legs should be considered as the diagnostic base. The veterinarian will flex and hold all or most of the joints on the leg in question. The veterinarian will hold the limb or limbs in a flexed position for about one to two minutes. The vet will then require the horse to "trot off" in hand. After the horse has trotted off in his exam, the veterinarian will assess and categorize the appearance of the "flexion test" and give it a "grade." In my experience, the cause of the lameness is not always readily obvious. I have had horses undergo a flexion test that unveiled a compensatory issue or even an area that became obvious only after a flexion test. Some veterinarians may choose to see a horse and rider combination working with the tack on as well and repeat the flexion test.

This is the basic exam that will determine any further diagnostics. If the veterinarian has questions about the flexion exam, they may want to utilize other methods of diagnostics to determine the horse's lameness issues.

As an aside: Some horses can present a bridle lameness, which means under working tack, they appear lame. This confusing lameness is usually rider-related, assuming we have ruled out faulty equipment and asymmetrical body imbalances of the horse. This lameness must be observed and commented on, as it is a legitimate lameness and must be brought to the rider's attention.

Nerve Blocks:

After the basic lameness exam, the vet may deem further diagnostics necessary. The idea of the nerve block is to determine and locate the actual area of injury. The vet will inject a "block" of an anesthetic-type drug that will numb the area in question. The veterinarian will then perform the basic flexion exam again. The block will make the area that is painful not hurt, and the horse will "appear" sound. This procedure will substantiate any lameness areas in question. Some veterinarians may require even more diagnostics; some may be satisfied with the results of this exam.

Radiographs are not usually used in a soft-tissue injury but may be used to rule out any bone-related lameness issues.

Ultrasound:

An ultrasound is the most common diagnostic for any soft-tissue areas in question. The ultrasound consists of a probe that emits high-frequency waves; the waves bounce off the tissues of the limb, are transmitted through a probe, and are then displayed on a viewing monitor. The monitor usually will have a keyboard, and the keyboard will have various tools for marking the location and size of the injury. Some of the more updated ultrasound machines can record the exam on a CD or DVD. Some of the older machines will utilize a printer that can record the image. This diagnostic will be repeated as often as the veterinarian requires. This is also how the vet will keep track of the healing process during a rehabilitation program as well.

THERMOGRAPHY:

This diagnostic tool detects inflammation in the entire body of the horse by recognizing areas that are holding heat. The areas of heat are represented on a Thermography scan as red (being the hottest), yellow, and orange. Cooler areas show up as blue. This technique can be used over multiple areas of the horse's body, for a variety of issues.

NUCLEAR SCINTIGRAPHY:

This form of locating inflammation within the horse involves using an injection of radioactive isotopes to locate areas of inflammation. The areas of inflammation will absorb more of the radioactive isotopes. A bone scan will read these levels, and they will be displayed as a picture; the areas of inflammation will be viewed with more isotopes around the injury site. One must realize that this involves an overnight stay at a clinic. Due to the nature of this procedure, it can be quite costly. It can be considered a good method of diagnostics after the horse is either not responding to a program or has not received a satisfactory answer as to an undetermined lameness.

There are other advanced methods of determining lameness as well; these are the most commonly used for soft-tissue injury diagnostics.

CHAPTER THREE
My Formula for Soft-Tissue Rehabilitation:

If the horse is off of work for one week, then he will need one week off for rest and the second week off for rehabilitation work.

And relative to the diagnosis, the following formula will follow:

2 weeks off of work, 4 weeks of rehab

1 month off of work, 2 months of rehab

Rehabilitation is defined as a process of restoring to good condition.

CAN I TURN OUT MY INJURED HORSE?

Does our partner horse not deserve this time off to heal?

If you can **guarantee** your horse will not play in turnout, then I wish you all the luck in the world. **I highly recommend hand-grazing**

and/or walking the horse for the first month until your veterinarian tells you otherwise. This is especially true for the performance horse; the horse that has a weekend job or casual job may be able to have a small turnout program. The only time I have ever viewed a horse being perfectly still was in a picture. This "jail time" could save you many months of future agony. You may hear words like "give him a gram of Bute, Banamine, DMSO, poultice, a few days off, no work, only walking, then back to work." Sometimes the advice of others may be the answer, but one must really educate oneself and realize the implications and healing time of a soft-tissue injury. Your veterinarian is the professional as to the best case program, and you know your horse the best. Work with the veterinarian and do not make hasty, unsupported decisions at any point during this time.

This program requires educated professional attention.

Relative Idea

When you have sprained your ankle—as we all have—think about how long it takes to really be back to 100 percent. One week, possibly two, sometimes longer? This is a soft-tissue injury, a twist, sprain, or strain. We did too much yard work, over-exercised at the gym, played a long game of tennis or golf, or even rode too much. Usually, we have overexerted our muscle strength, which causes stress on our ligaments and tendons. Our ligaments attach bone to bone; our tendons attach muscle to bone. So as we have tired and fatigued our large supportive muscles, our tendons and ligaments are still used without the support of the muscle strength. We can realize that we are a little sore, and usually take it easy for a few days. We may take an anti-inflammatory, ice our injury, use some Epsom salts in a bath, wrap our leg in an Ace bandage, and relax for a few days. About twenty-four hours later, we feel much worse, because now all the lactic acids that have been released from the broken-down muscle fibers are flying around our bodies. Now we are really sore—our "not-quite-right" feeling. Usually in a mild case of strain or sprain, we feel better in about five days. By the next two weeks, we barely are complaining of our weekend exploits, and are ready for the next round of overdoing life. But our muscle cells are still healing; they do not hurt but are not yet healed.

Our horses are similar. They realize they are a little sore and come out of the stall stiff and feeling not quite right. They may be a bit quieter that day; they keep working—or they don't, and then we grab the whip and spur! Because now we believe they are being difficult.

Even when they feel bad, they will still run down the fence line; they do not know how to stop. Some amount of thought really needs to be given to the work and rest load for the horse. I am not suggesting that all soft-tissue injuries occur from muscle fatigue, but many of them are from overwork. We, as riders and trainers, get a little greedy sometimes when we are trying to work through training issues. That happens to all of us—our determination to "make it better" sometimes takes over. So we must find that balance between exertion, building muscles, and resting; not always concentrating on collection, but realizing that collection develops from going easily and freely forward. By creating a swinging back and engagement of the hindquarters is how we achieve correct lightness and self-carriage—not through holding and resistance. We must remember as riders that just because we are having a hard time achieving a concept does not mean the horse is. These are dressage terms, but the ideas hold true to most riding disciplines. So the ideal training program would be combining forward exercises, bending and stretching exercises, and collected exercises, and incorporating them on separate days. If you work out and lift weights, you don't only do thigh squats every day with the same amount of weight. Why? Because the rest of your body will not properly develop the other vital supportive muscle groups. You will only set your body up to be susceptible to muscle fatigue and then injury. The same idea should be utilized for the program of the horse. The continual badgering to get a shoulder-in all week long is not going to get the horse to do the perfect shoulder-in. But if one can ride a correct ten-meter circle with rhythm, relaxation, and regularity, then this is the understanding of one of the basic foundations of all lateral work and a solid foundation to the development of the horse's training program.

We must never forget a proper warm-up and cool-down time as well, for any riding discipline.

Remember, it is many pieces of the horse's and rider's training that creates a beautiful movement or perfect performance.

WHAT YOU CAN DO BEFORE YOU RECEIVE VETERINARY HELP, IF YOU SUSPECT AN INJURY:

These are simple ideas for a non-traumatic injury; traumatic injuries will need immediate veterinary attention.

Making a basic assessment: You notice swelling and feel heat on a lower limb—the most important issue. Use both the front and back of your hand to feel the leg area; this helps for temperature accuracy. Repeatedly running your hand down the tendon will create heat. This can be confusing information when trying to assess a leg. Feel both legs of the pair as well, to compare the temperature. There are many other issues that can give the horse's leg a "fat" or "big" appearance as well: fungus, fever, and cellulitus, an infection that can cause mild swelling, skin sensitivity, as well the changing of the seasons can also cause the horse's legs to swell. Some horses' legs will swell during hot, humid weather and from continually stomping at the flies.

Is the horse lame in the walk or trot? Pick up his hoof like you are going to pick out his feet, and feel the leg; a very slight squeeze on the tendons will indicate pain. Be careful—he may pull the leg back quickly, especially if he is in pain. The swelling does not have to be extreme to be a serious issue.

If you can determine this on your own or there is a possible question of an injury, treat the inflammation very conservatively. If you have access to ice, use it in twenty-minute intervals, twenty minutes on the area in question, twenty minutes off. Some people use frozen bags of peas as a source of cold. Peas are very malleable and conform nicely around the leg. Wrap the entire bag around the leg with a polo wrap or track bandage. There are also many icing products available for humans that you can get at any local drug store, if you cannot get to a well-stocked tack store for your needs.

Ice packs are a good item to have in your emergency kit. These products will help to bring down any swelling. It is important not to put ice directly on the leg; you could possibly cause frostbite and destroy healthy tissue. If you do not have access to ice, use cold hose water twenty minutes on, twenty minutes off, as many times as you can during the day. This will be helpful, prior to a veterinary evaluation. Also, do not turn the horse out if there is suspicion of an injury.

NOTE: Do not wrap the horse's leg if you do not know how to or cannot wrap the horse because he is not used to being in standing leg wraps, and is also not used to being put into a stall with wraps on his legs.

If you need another non-invasive idea, take a handful of poultice and slop it on the inflamed leg area.

Take a hint from pottery class: Keep the horse's leg wet and keep a small pan of water near you when you are applying poultice. Wet your hands when you take a big clump of the clay out of the container and apply it to the horse's leg; use your pan of water frequently to dip your hands into. This will help keep the clay more workable as you spread it onto the injured or possibly injured area.

After you have cold hosed the horse's leg a few times during the day and if you can wrap the horse's leg, apply the poultice to the leg and use a paper towel or toilet paper around the poulticed area. "Touch" the paper with a little more water and it will stay on nicely. Paper towels are easy to work with; even easier to use is a roll of toilet paper. You can put a standing bandage over this. It replaces the older idea of the brown paper bag or grain bag to keep the poultice wet. If your vet cannot see your horse within the same day, this will help to start cooling the leg down and reduce the inflammation. It is also wise to keep some anti-inflammatory medicines in your medicine cabinet for just such a case. Your veterinarian can suggest some user-friendly medications that will not cause complications.

If you cannot wrap the horse's leg in bandages, make sure the leg remains somewhat wet. You can take handfuls of shavings from the stall and paste them to the poultice; this practice helps to hold the poultice in place for a while on a horse that does not handle standing wraps well. You must realize that your horse may end up with the poultice all over his face and body, and all over the stall by morning, especially if you need to put him in a stall using this concept. I usually put the poultice on the horse in the stall when I use this method, because I do not want him tracking poultice all over the place and not keeping the poultice on the injured leg. This idea is best for the young horse and for horses that are not used to confinement. Also, giving them some hay to eat will keep them occupied during this time.

The most important issue is to decrease the inflammatory process with ice or cold hosing. Do not use poultice on the leg and do not use any wrap if there is an open wound. This must be seen by the veterinarian. The only exception is a bleeding injury; in this event, a wrap or tourniquet is necessary.

These basic ideas are to assist and slow down the inflammation response prior to professional care. Your veterinarian cannot perform a diagnostic ultrasound until a large part of the inflammatory response has been decreased.

So to help your horse out immediately is to be an educated first responder. Hopefully your veterinarian can get to your barn within the day and help provide you with more information regarding your concerns.

Please remember, this is a serious injury, but it is not life-threatening unless it is a trauma. Other equine emergencies may take precedence over this veterinary issue especially if you veterinarian has a solely mobile practice.

This injury may also be discovered best by an equine clinic; they will have multiple types of diagnostic equipment. This is useful if you can travel with your horse, and continue to have undiagnosed lameness issues. This is especially important when you are in an area with limited equine veterinary access.

During the assessment, the veterinarian will give you the necessary medications and rehabilitation program you will need for the future and provide information as to when the horse should respond to a program. But always remember, the quicker you initially respond, the better position you are in for success. The more knowledge you have, the better you can be in every aspect of your life.

Life is not riding; riding is life. —R.K.

Chapter Four
Do you use a proctologist for podiatry?

I certainly hope the answer is no. The question reinforces my point that it is **imperative** that you locate a veterinarian who works with performance horses. Your local neighborhood good guy, kind-hearted Dr. Doolittle, cat, ferret, parrot, gerbil, and dog vet does not have the opportunities to see performance-horse injuries very often. He may be able to initially help control the inflammation and be your "primary care physician," but he should also respect the fact that experience is an undisputable factor. I have the highest regard for any person who has become a veterinarian. Their dedication, depth of knowledge, the little money they receive for a lengthy education and extraordinary time commitments are commendable. As trainers and riders, we all excel in certain areas of our life—showing, training, and management, running a successful business or getting our job done. So let the people with the most experience in the area of sport-horse injuries do what they do best. Find a veterinarian who deals with sport horses.

Call your local racetrack; find out from a hunter, jumper, dressage, combined training, Western reining, and barrel-racing organization; call anyone you know who has a performance-horse background and multiple injury experiences. Many of these injuries are vastly under-diagnosed and lead to a lifelong soundness struggle. These vets will probably be more expensive, because they are usually specialists who focus mostly on equine lameness. But you will pay more in the long run if your original diagnosis is not the best. A sport-horse veterinarian probably has quite a few horses he sees **daily** from sports-related lameness. The average horse veterinarian **may** have dealt with a tendon injury every other month. A racetrack veterinarian has a great deal of experience in speed-induced injuries. A jumper-and-hunter veterinarian has vast experience with concussion and stress-related injuries. A dressage veterinarian has training in diagnosing isometric, eccentric, and stress-related lameness. The saddle-seat veterinarian has to be very aware of the shoeing requirements and possible problems that can challenge the gaited horses. The combined-training veterinarian has "combined" issues, as does a veterinarian who deals with Western horses. So I cannot emphasize enough the importance of having a veterinarian who is trained and experienced in sport-horse injuries make this diagnosis. This may be more of a challenge for those who live in areas that are more remote and have limited sport horses.

Here are a few key points to keep in mind:

+ After the initial inflammation has been controlled or there is suspicion of a soft-tissue injury, you must get an ultrasound.
+ Make sure your veterinarian has a printer, CD, or can hard-copy the images. **You** need to keep a physical record, so you can compare the healing process and the activity of healing.
+ An ultrasound is the simplest and best diagnostic tool available. Make sure your veterinarian initially compares the **good leg and injured leg**. One needs to see what the healthy leg looks like, to give you a comparison of normal.
+ Make sure they **shave** the area they are to ultrasound. There are too many artifacts and oddities that can occur and create a misdiagnosis!
+ Make sure the veterinarian also has experience reading injury ultrasounds as well. It is not an easy task and requires a very skilled eye with multiple experiences. Ultrasound technicians for human patients go to school for two years specifically for reading ultrasounds.

Each leg is as individual as the horse it is attached to; a leg that looks strange on a particular horse may be perfectly normal for that horse. This is the best control you have as to what is normal and what is not. The diagnostic ultrasound will give you a cross-section of what the damaged tissue looks like. It can tell you the extent of the damage you have, and the size of damaged tissue. Normal tendon tissue has elastic-like quality; this makes sense in light of the job the tendons and ligaments do for the body. The tendons and ligaments need to elongate or stretch and receive concussion for the movements of the horse; they also need to spring back.

When this tissue becomes inflamed, it takes on the appearance of an undefined mosaic under an ultrasound reading. The tendon tissue appears spread out, and the cells are filled with fluid and swollen. Some of the ultrasound scans will even contain black spots; this must be taken very seriously, as this could possibly mean there is a hole or tear in the tissue. The normal tendon tissue is a nicely organized, tightly woven mosaic with clear definition to the cell walls. There is an amount of color ranging from white to grays and black. There are nice separations between all the tendons, and your vet should explain to you what you are observing. Remember, the ultrasound image is a "sideways view" into the tendons and ligaments. Not all black spots mean a hole in the tendon, so do not panic. Not all white lines are scar tissue. This is where a trained eye is imperative. There will be some black and some white in the imaging; these can possibly be the bones, veins, and blood vessels, and spaces that naturally occur in the structure of the limb.

Correct diagnostics are extremely important. Ultrasounds need to be done approximately every thirty days, until the healing tissue remains at a constant; some tissue will never look good again but may remain at a constant appearance. That may be the best the tissue will get in appearance. Some tissue may actually stop healing and will require another veterinary consultation as to what steps to take next. Usually on the **best** ultrasound during rehabilitation, you are only looking at juvenile tissue; this is not workable tissue. But this is a very positive sign of healing!

Wait at least one more month and stick with your program. Get another ultrasound; if you are happy with the news this month, you will be ecstatic next month.

Before you begin your trot program and your canter program, I recommend ultrasounds, just to track your progress and make sure you still have the green light for work. Your goal with the ultrasound scans is to keep viewing the healing process and to try to prevent scar tissue from limiting the amount of flexibility the tendons and ligaments will have. Scar tissue makes the injured tissue more rigid and less stretchy, which can be career-ending to some horses if the rest-and-rehabilitation program is not very aggressive. Some scar tissue and rigidity will happen because of the nature of the injury and the healing process, but it is the effort we are putting in to increase our odds of healthy tissue growth.

Above all, be realistic about healing time. If your horse is off for a month, that means it will be two months before you are back to easy work. If it requires six months off, realize that you have a year before you are back to true work. You must understand that you are basically conditioning the horse back into a working life. Don't simply hope and pray; take the time and be smart. Recognize your injury, cry your heart out, and deal with your dance partner. **You will be successful.** If you cannot handle the task, walk away and let someone do this for you—a professional. There are many very reputable lay-up and rehabilitation farms that have very solid programs.

You may choose to sell your horse because rehabilitation is too much to do by yourself or you do not want to pay expenses for a horse you cannot ride for a year. Figure this out quickly; your opportunity to have success is directly proportional to your emotional limitations. Work through your feelings and put your horse in the best-case scenario for him. You may decide to put him out in the field, because you "cannot deal with it." This answer to me is tragic, especially if the horse can have a future based on a program; then it is worth the time. You have an obligation to your horse. In an older horse, other decisions may be acceptable, such as retirement, as long as the horse is comfortable and can move without great struggle or pain.

You may say to yourself that you cannot make a decision as to your horse's condition, but you have—*no decision* is still a decision. You must accept the fact that their careers may be limited when they recover. I was tortured by this as a professional, but here is the conclusion I came to: Every day I would feel I was the prison warden, and Buddy was out with me or trapped in his stall. If I did not show up, he stayed looking at the walls. If I did go to the barn, he got an hour or two of attached freedom. So I said to myself, "Here is the reality: You cannot afford to replace him; if you turn him out and he hurts himself again, that is it. He will be a cripple, limited in any future career. Every day you will have to wake up and look at him, wondering *if I kept him inside and stayed very focused for one year, could I have made a difference?* What is one year in a lifetime? The second question became, Could I handle the guilt that *I chose to release him to his own devices?* Then I crippled my horse or I have to put him down, because I couldn't "handle it." The answer was: "No way."

So I told myself this story every time I thought of giving up. Another horse I had for a two-year rehabilitation was young and untrained; I must admit I did give up. I had spent seven months resting and walking this untrained four-year-old. I was told after this rest time, he was a surgical candidate. I had given my best to this horse, and to hear that I was look-ing at two-year rehabilitation on a very talented, untrained horse put me into a very trying time emotionally and professionally. I must admit I did crumble; it took me about a month to get my energy back together for this horse. I had spent every day for seven months with this guy, and thought I was looking at a work program. This horse almost killed me; he dragged me on my belly and side at least fifty feet one day and I wanted to let him go in the worst way, but I couldn't. I couldn't let all of that time and work go running around the arena. I knew he would eventually stop after all the ground work I had done. I saw the light at the end of the tunnel and soldiered on. He needed me, and I knew this horse would be okay; I needed to get myself focused again and do my program.

If you can afford to get a new horse, then that may be the best decision for you and your horse. If you cannot … you choose. These are your hard and real facts, and this is now your reality.

"But this is just a horse. I have stuff to do. Kids, husband, taxes, my world, my life! This … I have no time for." The choice be-comes priorities and obligations.

Chapter Five
A Plan

After the initial diagnosis and the actual reality of exactly how your life is going to change settles in, you need to have a plan. You cannot possibly conceive of the time commitment and the physical therapy demands you are going to face. You are the average person; you have a life, a family, and a job. So if you are not willing or able to truly dedicate yourself as the healer, *get some help*. There are rehabilitation farms, and people who get paid to rehabilitate horses—a very good groom at your barn or a local training facility. It is important to find a person who has experience and knowledge of rehabilitation with horses and is a very good horse handler. These are the qualities that they or you must have for this job. Do not be cheap and try to pawn this job off on an overeager teen or a soft-hearted friend. It is a difficult and dangerous job.

I know of a tale about a lovely young teenage girl in my town of Jupiter, Florida who was unintentionally and tragically killed on her family's front lawn by her stall-bound horse. She was, to my knowledge, given no indication of what her love—her horse—was to become after a significant stall-rest injury. This was a tragic and preventable story, but a reality for other horsemen and veterinarians to appreciate. The severity of this injury time and the knowledge that must be provided to horse owners and handlers during this time is significant for their safety, as well as the horse's.

It also may help to remove you from the equation, especially if you are not able to handle what will quickly become intense. Your horse also does not need to have your anxieties to deal with as well as his while he is healing.

THE EQUINE PERSONALITY

Now let's take a look at our horse: an animal that does not understand and cannot rationalize "taking it easy." We are the primary caretakers, the only ones who can help our friend make a full recovery. So to us, two weeks to heal needs to be thought of as one month off of true work. I am sure many of you may say I am too conservative. For every week off, it takes one week to build the horse back to fitness. So again we do our math: two weeks of rest, two weeks of recovery.

One month down time. This also may mean

NO TURNOUT *for the entire process and possibly the horse's lifetime.*

I cannot overemphasize the importance of total rest and total controlled movements. I **know** you are thinking, *my horse is going to get crazy, he will kick the walls down,* and you are right. They are athletes with competitive lifestyles, jobs, and routines. But it is better that they are crazy in a twelve-by-twelve space than tearing across their paddock and becoming a permanent cripple. This is especially true for sport horses. If a horse is a really tough patient, pet, or casual companion, the veterinarian may allow turnout in a very small paddock or hospital stall, a turnout paddock not much larger than a sixteen-by-sixteen area where the horse can "go out" without actually being uncontrolled. If your facility has in-and-out stalls, you can do what we did, and make a small turnout for a young horse, with veterinary approval. This actually made a significant difference in the horse's mental attitude during his two-year program. He was never unsupervised during his turnout time; we gave him hay to eat outside, and he was actually much quieter to handle and less dangerous. Again, you really have to know what kind of horse you are dealing with. Remember, horses are of three mindsets: flight, fright, or fight, and we do not want any of these natural instincts to become out of control.

Creating a routine is primary. Stay the course, and don't give up on a whim. Instead of feeling bad, breaking your heart, feeling cruel, and calling yourself a bad horse owner, think of your animal, stay with the treatment routine, and get to work. If you choose to do this yourself, your horse needs you to walk him. Work with the barn manager and see if you can have a different stall, something quieter or where the horse can see activity; it depends on what your horse likes to see. Many, many horses spend their entire lives without being turned out, and only working. It is **okay,** they will adjust; it is only temporary in the grand scheme of life. Give them another job description.

ROUTINE IDEAS

Keep as much of the horse's daily routine the same as possible so they can keep their jobs. Walk them before, after, or around turnout time, **after** the other horses have gone out, and **only** if the other horses are quiet. Some horses will be better at a more quiet time if you are at an active barn. Find some good grass for them to eat. Even go in their old pasture with them and hand-graze for as much time as you have. If you only have access to the arena, walk … walk … walk. The first ten minutes of each day's activity are usually the worst in terms of the horse's attitude and behavior. **Be careful.**

Horses do very well with a routine. If possible, try to keep them thinking they still have the same job. Some horses will do better at work time if they have another horse in the arena or work area with them, while some may use it as an excuse to play and be naughty; some even become defensive around other horses. A young horse that I had for rehabilitation had been very threatened when the other horses worked in the arena with him; he would put his ears back and lunge at the other horses! He would even walk tentatively and cautiously. When he was alone, he walked normally and with conviction.

These are herd animals. This horse knew he was hurt and weak, and he felt threatened by the other horses. It took me a little bit to interpret this behavior. He worked best alone, with a pony or an older horse. You will need to put some time into understanding behavior and making a routine that works for you and your horse. This is the time to use your creativity. Please be advised not to get *overly* creative, however. If the

way to have control of the horse as well. The capture chain or first idea prevents the halter from twisting into the horse's eye, and seems to offer a more uniform reprimand. You only tighten the chain when the horse is naughty; other than that, the chain lies softly on their nose. Make sure your halter fits your horse, and is snapped on or buckled properly. Make sure you have a throat latch; a grooming halter will not do. Choose either a good-quality leather or nylon halter. Attaching the lunge line properly will hopefully prevent the horse from getting unmanageable, but I also must contradict myself. Some horses can get defensive and aggressive when they have a chain over their nose. So, your individual plan must be in your and your horse's best interest.

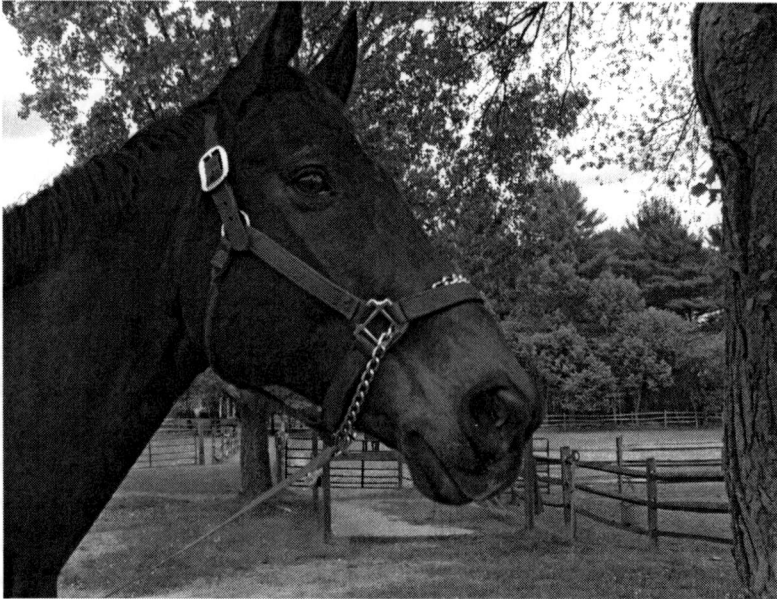

Please, never make a loop in a chain lead, attaching it back to itself and attaching it to the ring on the under part of the halter. This is the most dangerous way anyone could ever lead a horse. It is extremely dangerous because the horse can die. Here is what can happen: They can get their leg through the chain loop and the halter, panic, flip over, and break their neck. Don't **ever** do this in handling any horse. If you do not utilize the chain properly on this type of lead line, then you need to buy another lead line.

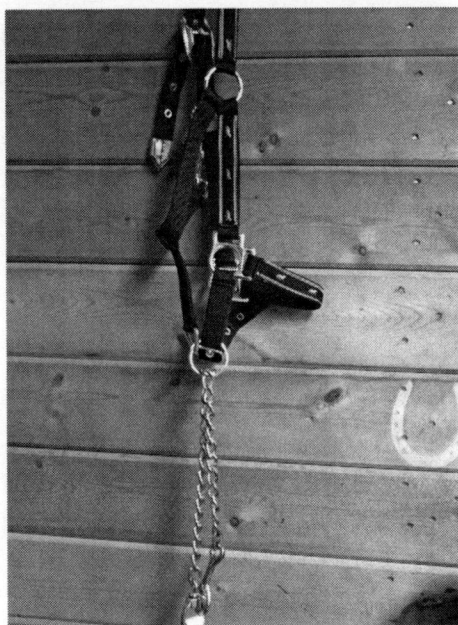

Bad Chain Idea

I prefer to use a cotton **lunge line with a chain shank.** Because this is what I know:

I guarantee your horse standing on his hind legs is longer than the lead line you are holding that you *think* is a good idea. I know that the leg he will kick out at your head is longer than the lead line you are holding as well. I know *they will scare* the poop out of you with their antics. I know this not because I am psychic, but because I do know horses, *and it will happen* to you in some way, shape, and form. Here is a simple test: Take your lead line and measure the length of the horse's hind leg and entire body, including the neck and head. If you have to double the lead line to measure, then it is not long enough to handle the horse safely.

There is a halter that I found in a Western tack store that worked really well without force, but from acupressure points. The halter works by knots on the acupressure points of the horse's face. The pressure provides control without punishment. Learn how to put this halter on properly, and make sure your lead is the correct length. I found a respectable difference when I used this halter. But you cannot use the chain shank lead as described when you use this halter, and I still recommend a long line.

I also carry a whip or riding bat with me as well. I have found myself in many predicaments where I was very glad I had carried that whip with me. Even if I used it only once, it was worth carrying every day.

You will need a very good pair of *leather* gloves, not fabric riding gloves, a glove made of leather. Riding gloves are made of fabric that tears and rips. The goatskin leather glove is soft and may be a good option. Leather is tough; your hands are not.

Here are some handling ideas to keep in mind:

- **Don't let go of your horse.** No matter what happens (unless you are knocked out and absolutely have to) you must be the anchor. Worst-case scenario: **You will get dragged.** This may be better then having your horse gallop at full speed down the farm's paved driveway with the lunge line trailing dangerously behind him. Establish your ground manners! The horse must know and respect the word "WHOA."

- **Use a paddock when you graze him** if you do not fully trust your horse in hand. I also suggest not getting too close. Let your horse have about six feet or more, and try to stay around his shoulder area and keep his back end away from your front end. If and when your horse decides to rear and buck—and he will—you will realize you need to move with your horse. The horse's shoulder is the safest place to be; that puts you out of the way of the flying back hooves. But be careful that the front-end hooves do not come above your head as well. Some horses like to strike out when they get excited. I carry a whip with me for unexpected behaviors.

- **Give yourself room** to step back and be safe if they bounce, kick out, rear, or whatever else they will do for a minute; catch your breath and continue walking. I reprimand my horses for this, but you must appreciate and have an understanding as to their behavior as well.

- **Do not let other folks distract your attention;** others may want to talk to you, you may want to use your cell phone and want to socialize during this time, because you may see it as a casual vacation. I suggest always having your eyes on your horse. YOU are all they have at this point in time, and you need to be aware of all situations that could potentially become dangerous. Horses are scorekeepers; they know how many mistakes you are making before you even realize you are in trouble.

The poor guys are hurt and frustrated with their changed lifestyle. So if you have a well-trained and controlled horse on the ground, you can let him **bounce** safely, while you remain calm. Screaming and yelling at him for exploding every once in a while will just make him more excited or scared. If you are not careful with these moments, you can get in big trouble **FAST**. If they are allowed to get too crazy, they will really take advantage of you, and now you cannot control them at all. When the time comes that you can ride them, this will only get much worse, and more dangerous.

So with extreme caution I say this: You must have **absolute** control. If your horse is not a great longer, if he pulls, drags, pushes, and rubs on you, and if he does not lead perfectly, **I mean PERFECTLY**, and if you do not feel confident in your horse-handling ability, **do not take any chances;** be very strong with your expectations and corrections. If you cannot be this type of horseman, find someone or someplace that can.

This "bouncing" is not ideal, but it will happen, and it is better than having uncontrolled running; remember, you must **try** to control all of the movement of your horse.

Finally, be aware of your surroundings. Make sure your horse does not lure you to let him graze under any low overhangs or fences, or get you blocked into a corner. Be aware, and always have enough room to avoid getting stuck in a dangerous predicament. This way, you can assess a situation instead of being part of it, and if your horse rears, leaps, kicks at you, or bucks, you are clear. Again, if this does happen, **try not to let go of him.** Many of our horses have rather catlike abilities, injured or not. I only mention being farther away because I find I have the time to get away from them if I give myself an extra six feet to begin with. Be aware that these guys can whirl, kick, rear, buck, leap on top of you, pull, fly backward, and a variety of other very impressive acrobatics you have never seen before in your once-familiar friend. Reprimand them; they cannot do this. As hard as it may be to reprimand your ever-so-frustrated horse, he cannot be naughty. Otherwise you will allow and create the most horrible and very hard-to-fix demon seed. Be firm and keep control at all times. Do not get panicky, scared, and stupid. Keep a clear head and focus on the job at hand. Now you are becoming a horseman instead of a horse owner. Re-assess your position during these times, and determine if you are still the best person for this rehabilitation time.

When you are doing any in-hand work, be sure to not let him step on or over the lead as you hand-walk and graze him. Do not multitask and catch up on your phone calls when you are handling your rehabilitation horse. **Hang up the cell phone, take off your ipod** and give your undivided attention to your circumstances.

> Things you will need:
> gloves
> helmet
> whip or riding crop
> sneakers and riding footwear
> a good halter and longe line
> a calendar and pen
> a watch
> any type of cooling lotion, poultice, or gel
> leg wraps or standing wraps
> boots or polo wraps for support while working
> a program of routine and nutritional support
> a good constitution
> a large amount of time
> a large amount of patience

I was able to take my older horse to his favorite roll spot in his paddock. (Ask your veterinarian if this is a possibility for you. The action of getting up and down may be too stressful on some injuries.) You may find the horse will like to have a roll in the dirt. Some horses will just drop and roll anywhere. Just let them have that roll, and be careful not to get the lunge wrapped around the legs or around their necks give them a little extra line and space. Oh, and don't overreact if this happens. **Go with them** in this situation; let them roll, keep calm, and use your voice and the training you hopefully have established by now. Keep a treat in your pocket, just in case they get fresh after they get up from their roll! I think every horse knows the snap of a carrot. The first ten minutes out of the stall are often the most terrible in terms of reactions. They seem to really be reactive after coming out of the stall, ready to have their thirty minutes of freedom. After the first ten minutes, they seem to settle a bit, but do not hold me to this at all. This is merely my personal observation and experience.

If they can graze, great! Find the best grass. If they can't, then make them walk, very businesslike, very actively. Do not allow them to have a crazy, dangerous walk that could involve them trying to hurt you! This businesslike pace should be the pace of choice. Remember to keep the horse's shoulder in front of you and be careful not to let them swing their bodies around you. They will settle down if you are very diligent about their program. Do not be afraid to call it quits on any particular day either. Some days are not going to be days when you can do your normal program. Windy, cool days, change of seasons, weaning of young horses, breeding days, and any day that changes the energy of the farm environment is a day that needs to be approached differently than a NORMAL day. And if you need to get fit and lose weight, you will have the ultimate program. I guarantee it! Twice a day for at least thirty to forty-five minutes of walking and hand-walking your horse is the best way to lose weight. Never mind the emotional stress! This rehabilitation time really makes your life change.

I preferred being on my older horse's back during his rehabilitation; I could not keep up with my horse's enormous walk. My horse is seventeen hands high, and his size added to his energy level. My preference was in the saddle on his back. I find some horses are better when they are in their working tack, even when I am just hand-walking them. Be aware that your horse will get spoiled. He depends on you for *every ounce of freedom* now. So do not forget to apply the ground rules every day. The horse has to remember who the boss is, regardless. And remember, every day is not the same as the one before. Your horse may have been calm and quiet for two days in a row while you were hand-walking him. But at any given time, he **may** explode with unfamiliar energy.

Always be prepared and aware that this can and will happen.

CHAPTER SEVEN
Medications

This is a reality you may face: Veterinary consultation **is imperative.** The usual medications prescribed by the veterinarian are initially anti-inflammatory, which could be a steroid-based drug. Azium and Naquazone are some common names, so be aware if there are laminitis issues in the horse, Cushing's disease, or if the horse is a stallion or a pregnant mare. This could cause serious complications.

A second course of medications may follow, a series of NSAIDS (non-steroidal anti-inflamatories)—Banamine, Bute, and Naproxen, to name a few. Ask your veterinarian what these drugs are best used for. The drugs previously mentioned help reduce the inflammation of the leg. I recommend staying with the ice or cold hose and poultice routine for at least thirty-six to forty-eight hours after the initial injury. It may be necessary to keep the horse on this program with or without drugs for an extended timeframe until the leg no longer displays any signs of heat and sensitivity. Make sure you purchase a non-irritating poultice, one the horse can live in as well!

When the time is right, you will no longer need drugs for the initial injury. Now you may need to think of drugs for safety reasons. As your horse starts to feel better, he will start to get fresh. Hopefully, since the initial down time, you have re-established some new rules and have a well-behaved horse. **It is very wise to use this time well.** I cannot express this strongly enough. Do not be casual and think this is a vacation; it is the *most intense* time you will ever spend with your horse. I realize I am repeating myself, but it is necessary for my readers to be reminded of certain topics again.

The reality will be that some horses will need a long-term calming drug or mild tranquilizer. There are limited options; a long-term anti-psychotic like Reserpine, in my experience, is the most successful. You must monitor the dosage of this drug, as it can give a horse diarrhea. There is a loading dose, but some horses will be fine on a much smaller dose. Reserpine can also be injected into the horse; I prefer the pill form, because I can control the dosage as needed. An injection is limited, as once it is in, it cannot be taken out or adjusted, and if it does not work, you only find that out when you are in trouble. Some veterinarians may find the use of Reserpine controversial as well. DO NOT combine any drug therapies unless the veterinarian approves of this. Tranquilizers like Acepromazine and Rompum can be helpful, but these are not guaranteed. They require a knowledgeable person an educated handler, and a calm environment. Acepromazine and Rompum can backfire dangerously, and Acepromazine and Reserpine used in the wrong combinations can kill a horse. If one chooses a daily injectable drug, the horse will become aware of getting his "shot"; this can be dangerous, as the anticipation can make the horse anxious and lash out. If this becomes a daily routine, you must be aware of the side effects of long-term drug use, gastric ulcers are sometimes discovered during long-term drug use. Stallions and some geldings should not have Acepromazine, as it can affect their organs of fertility.

Veterinary input is imperative with any medicinal use.

It is also good to keep something in your program that supports the horse's digestive system. Because of the emotional stress and the long-term drug use as factors of your rehabilitation program, one must consider additional therapies. Brand names like Gastroguard, Ulcerguard, and Success are great intestinal support. Cimetidine is useful as well. There are also many natural cures; for example aloe juice, sodium bicarbonate (baking soda), and the use of digestive clays are other natural remedies as well. Basically, any kind of probiotic/ulcer product should be considered. Long-term use of Acepromazine, Banamine, Bute, and any NSAIDS can aggravate ulcers or even cause them. If antibiotics are required, one should definitely consider some alternative intestinal support. These are just other issues to be aware of. Do not go out and buy everything under the sun and overdo your horse's rehabilitation program from panic; just allow yourself to be educated. You have quality time on your hands now. Watch and see how your horse reacts to his new lifestyle. You may not need to use any alternative methods to calm and quiet him. Remember, if handling the horse becomes an issue, it is for your safety and his. Re-injuries take longer to heal than the initial ones. **Your personal injuries are forever.** You must realize all the time you will lose if you are not safe in your management program. As the exception to the rule, some horses are fantastic and will be troopers, handling down time very well and without any incident.

The homeopathic and natural aids can work very well—Rescue Remedy, Quietex, Quiescence, and B' Calm. Each horse is different; you may need to do some trial and error, and discuss the program with a professional. You will either say to yourself *this works* or *it does not,* in a matter of minutes during a session. Epsom salts can also have a calming effect when given orally, but in a closely monitored dose. The choice of magnesium-based supplements can really make a horse loose in his stools, which can lead to diarrhea and potentially dehydration. Calm'Em by Finishline is a magnesium-based product that I found helped my horse stay calm and focused. More recently, I used a Chinese herbal product called Shen Calm from a DVM in Reddick, Florida. You must get this product through a veterinarian, though. I had good success with this product.

Chapter Eight
Bandaging
Should You or Shouldn't You?

If you do not know how to do a supportive standing wrap, you will become the best wrapper in the world when this whole event is over. Some horses will not be able to tolerate this, but those handlers who can utilize this information will be able to incorporate these ideas into their program.

Wrapping the horse's legs gives the limbs support. Remember, the injury just took one leg away from your horse, and now the remaining three will be compensatory. Ligaments and tendons take a long time to heal, primarily because of the very slow blood supply that is in the tissue and gets to the tissue. So you need every opportunity to encourage healing. Wrapping also assists to stabilize a weakened limb. When you wrap the legs, you need to wrap both legs—whether the front pair or the back legs, you must wrap the pair. Again, I will contradict myself, because too many horses have made me a liar. Some horses, in my experience, will only accept a single wrap on the injured leg.

I prefer to use the firm support wrap with the foam on the inside; they are a thinner bandage, and I feel I can really control the application of the bandage better. You can use the pillow ones too, but my opinion is that they do not stay up as well. I also prefer an elastic-based track wrap.

The flannel wraps seem to require some amount of pulling, and I do not like pulling on the tendons or ligaments at all. I like flannels for shipping and protection, but prefer elastic track wrappers for injury support. I also like the Velcro attachments versus the use of safety pins, for obvious reasons.

I recommend twelve hours at the most in standing wraps and poultice. Please remember, unless this is a more traumatic injury that involves lacerations and sutures, bandaging requirements should be discussed with your veterinarian and will vary.

If your horse likes to chew at his wraps, here are a few ideas: Hot sauce, liquid soap, and any of the no-chew products you can buy at your local tack store may help. Many of these products that you can put on the bandages may contain capsicum, the stuff that makes chili peppers hot. These products will burn on contact the mucous membranes of the horse, his mouth and nose ... and yours too! So handle these products with caution and even wear vinyl gloves when applying. If this burns the horse's mouth, he hopefully will learn not to mess with his wraps. But be advised—you do not want your horse kicking at the burning on his injured leg, or frustrated by his burning nose!

- You may need to buy a bib or muzzle cage for your horse if he is very naughty and bandages are mandatory.
- **In a non traumatic injury if your horse truly cannot deal with wraps,** he will do more damage to himself trying to get them off than the wraps will be helpful. If possible at this point, don't wrap the leg; it **is not worth the repercussions of the horse's frustrations.**

If you do not know how to bandage, find someone with experience who can teach you. Some vets may not know how to do a performance horse standing wrap very well, especially if they do not do it every day. A groom from a show barn or the racetrack is usually quite experienced. Wrapping is an art unto itself. If you do not wrap your horse correctly, here is the harsh reality: You will make a bandage bow—another soft-tissue injury, created from too much pressure on the tendon, and the tendon sheath enlarges and bows out. This event will quickly become another downward spiral of frustrations. The wraps need to be secure but not tight. You should be able to get a finger comfortably into them. It is imperative not to twist the wraps in any way. Do not let the wrap slide around the leg as you put on the flannel or track bandage. Support the tendons as you work, and do not pull them at all. Place them around the leg. Also get wraps that fit your horse's leg. If your barn buddy has a pony and you have a seventeen-hand warm-blood, chances are their cannon bones are different sizes. It is in your best interest to invest in a set or two of quality standing wraps, for your own needs.

Basic Standing Wrap Bandaging

This method is good for any injury between the knee and fetlock area or the hock and fetlock. Your wrap and bandage lengths will vary depending on the length of your horse's cannon bone. Most tack stores have a supply of sizes.

1. (Assuming left foreleg.) Always work the bandages from the inside of the leg to the outside. Start on the cannon bone, placing the bandage between the knee and fetlock joint. Hold the wrap securely in place with your left hand while the right hand unrolls the bandage across the tendons. Do not pull, twist, or allow the wrap to become uneven on the leg. If you start the bandage in a firmly rolled position, the standing bandage will unroll better as you work.

2. Secure the back of the bandage with your right hand as you bring it across the cannon bone again; this helps prevent pulling and twisting. You can also feel the tension you are creating as you wrap.

3. I place my track wrap *into* the top quarter of my standing bandage; I prefer this method. It helps keep the track wrap secured. I also start my wrap in the upper middle section of the bandage; I wrap down to the fetlock and then return to the top of my bandage where the wrap ends. **This is a personal preference**.

4. As you start your wrap, make a complete wrap to secure the initial track wrap. I then go down halfway with the wrap and continue in halves as I continue down the leg and then when I have about a quarter of the underlying bandage remaining, I

start to go back up the leg, taking care not to pull. This way, I have a smooth wrap placement.

5.   I always end with a little of the bandage showing, about an eighth to a quarter inch on the top and bottom of my bandages. If you leave too much on the top and bottom, you may risk the wrap having too much pressure in a smaller area, and also offering a temptation for the horse to pull.

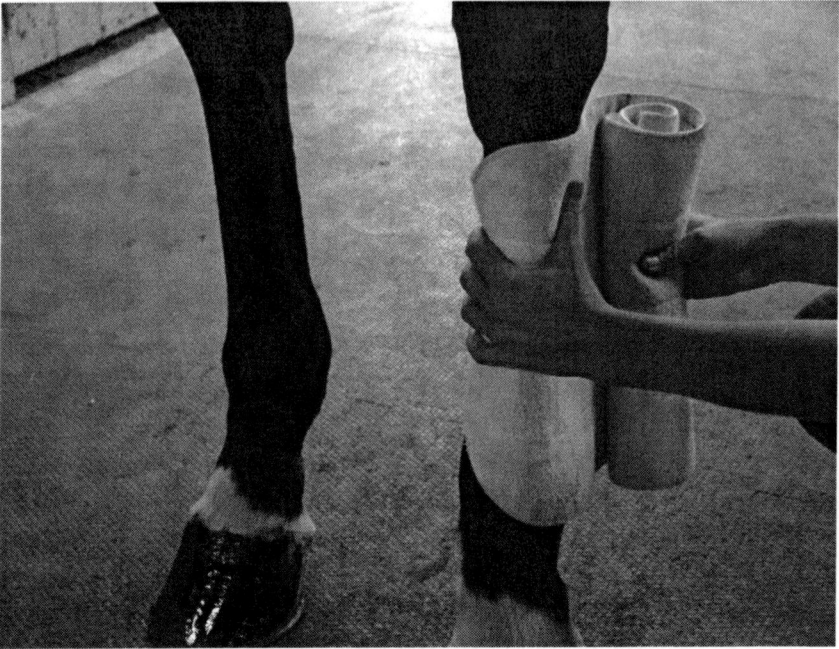

Place standing Bandage on cannon bone

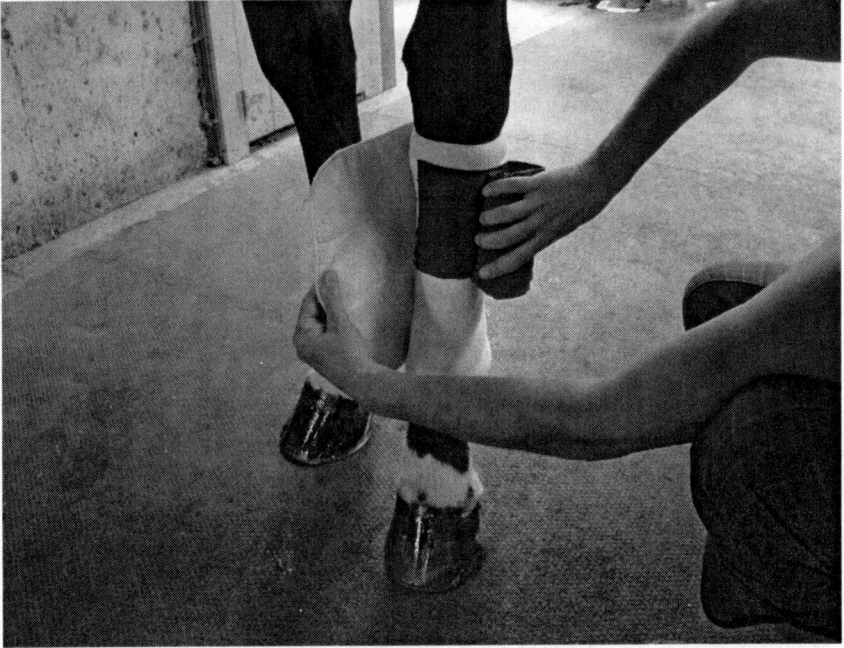

Place track wrap into the end of the standing bandage

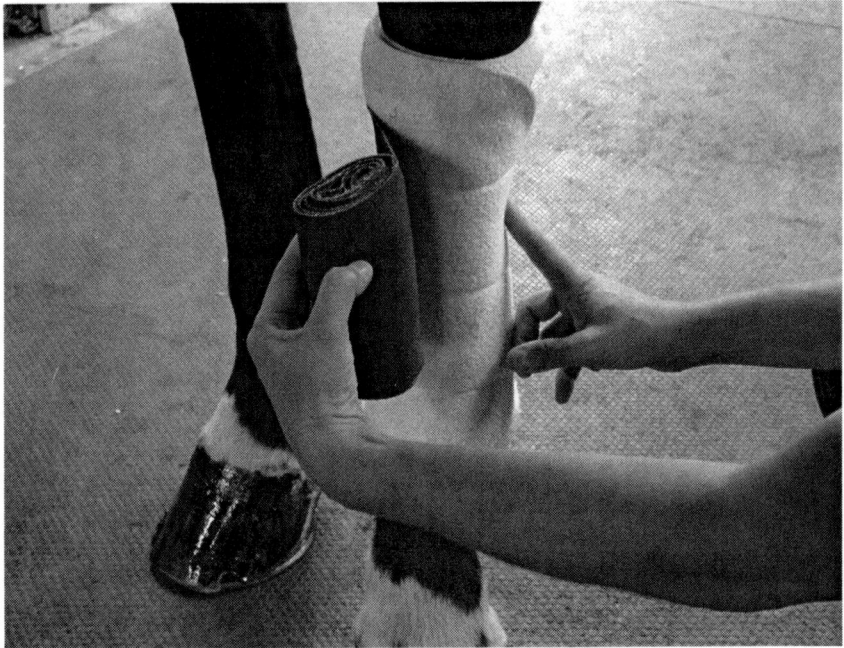

Continue

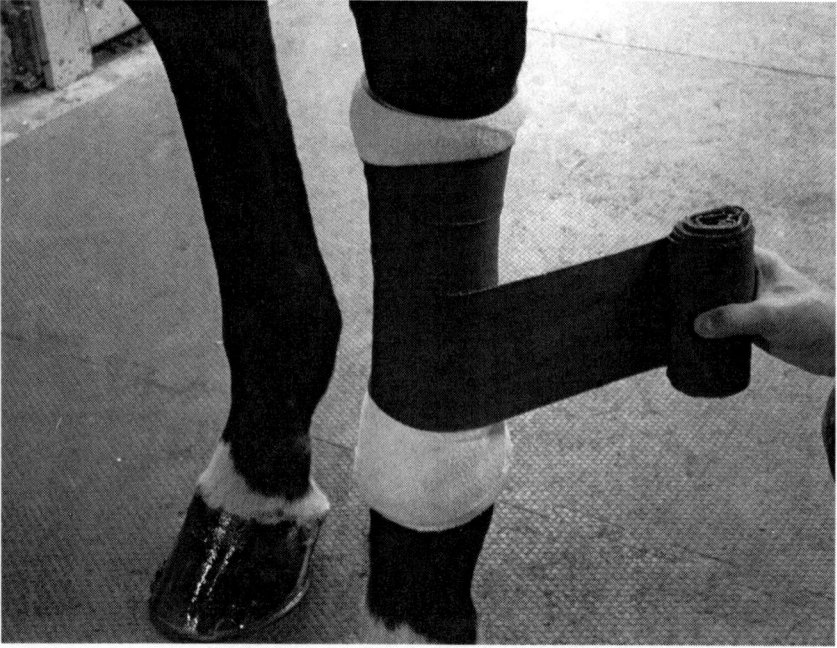

Continue in halves with the track wrap

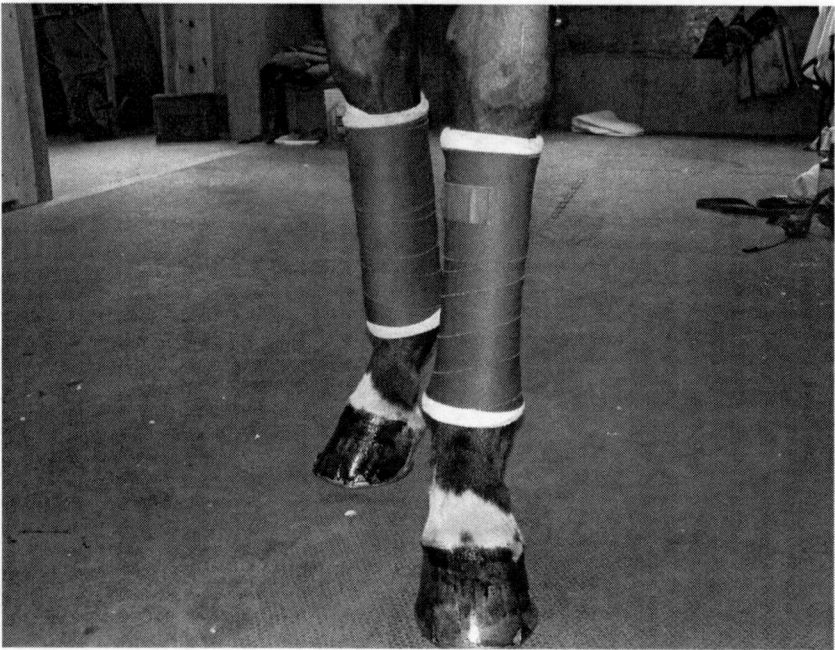

WHAT ELSE WILL I LEARN IN THIS TIME?

Some horses may develop some bad habits, such as wall-kicking, cribbing, weaving, and wood-chewing. I can suggest a few ideas. Move the horse to a quieter stall, possibly an end stall with a window; this gives him something to watch but not something to get anxious about. Your horse will dictate if he is better with stimuli or with quietness. You may need to find a stall that has fewer stimuli, but with some action, so he can at least be part of the daily events. If the horse becomes a wall-kicker, I can suggest padding the walls with rubber mats, typical of the ones used on the stall floors. You can screw the mats to the lower half of the stall walls, and when the horse kicks, he hits the padded wall first and this helps prevent any future leg injury. Kicking chains may be a possibility, but we must remember we are dealing with a leg injury; our resources can be limited.

If the horse becomes a "weaver," and starts rocking from side to side in front of the door, the more time out of the stall he can have, the better. This vice does not help the injured leg either. If the horse starts to crib, placing his teeth on something and sucking in air, there are many devices and products on the market that help curb this pattern of behavior. Horses that become wood-chewers will also respond best by keeping their minds tired; some people have success with a horse ball or horse toy that keeps the injured horse entertained. Toys have their place, but can also make a horse frustrated and more obsessed as well.

Everything will compound rapidly during the days of recovery. Try to do things correctly and with discipline; try to keep the horse mentally calm at this time, but do not go out and buy every toy ever created for the horse. Over-stimulation can be a very bad thing as well. It creates unneeded energy and more frustration. Most injured horses are very content to be left quietly in a stall, especially when they are resting and recovering.

I need to continue to remind you of this. Because we want so badly for our horse to be healthy and the way he was before, and for us to have that "fun" again with our friend.

So now go ahead and cry, scream, pitch a fit, get drunk, get mad, and then stop feeling sorry for yourself. Take all your knowledge and expertise and use it. Get ready for how much more you will learn about your horse and how you can help him. More information and questions than you ever could imagine will now come into your life. Be grateful for the knowledge you will receive from this experience. You may get depressed or cry or beat up on your friends and family emotionally, and feel you are somewhere between insanity and a nervous breakdown. This is okay. You only love your horse and you are being tested to the ultimate limit of that relationship. You *can* make it through this. Tell your loved ones they need to love you more. They do not have to understand; and that is okay, because they won't. And if you have a useless relationship, now is the time to see the light. You need a support system and friends who are there for you, and they need to and will appreciate this unfamiliar time. This is emotionally important during this rehabilitation time, because this is a part of what makes you who you are; what all your folks love about you. Share your trials with them. Hug, make dinner, or go out (if you are not exhausted); ask them to just understand that this is what makes you happy and this is the way of life for an equine enthusiast. For anyone to question, to argue, and to make you feel more isolated and fight with you is not going to change anything or make the stress any better; a team effort will be the best and allow this time to become much more successful. Now is the time to ask your partners for unconditional love and acceptance of the demands this personal situation requires. This is a much healthier approach to your entire program for you and your horse.

"Riding is life," and life is riding if you are a horseman.

Depression does not surface only through crying all the time. It can manifest into many a personality change, physical pain, and emotional instability. I have lived there threefold, and I hope to share with my readers some support. Every day, I would wake up and say to myself, "We have the opportunity to wake up every day and make it different than the day before." Every day I knew I was making a difference in my horse's future.

Find a good listener, or find ten. Just keep it together and keep marking those days off the calendar until the next ultrasound. This is most accurate for an individual private owner who has one horse. Trainers and those with multiple horse responsibilities will not have as many issues with this area. This may be helpful information for trainers and the like as to the emotional issues individual clients may be facing.

Learning is an active process, and essentially the responsibility of the learner.

CHAPTER TEN
Environment

I am sure most of us can say we feel better when the days are sunny and warm. The same is true of our horses. We layer our clothes in the cold, eat more food, and usually are not quite as active. We do not drink as much water, and it takes us longer to get things done. As our horse is faced with his injury, all factors must be considered. Environment must be thought of as one of these factors. When it is cold, our bodies utilize our energy to keep our temperature normal and our basic body functions working properly; we utilize our energy for exercise or work. When we are injured or ill, our bodies go into super survival mode, and that energy gets used to heal us. This is quite a large amount of energy consumption added on to our basic body function demands. Cold weather also can bring mental changes to your horse. Horses get excited in the cold weather; I think all horse owners will agree on that. There are the additional factors of snow falling from the roof of the indoor arenas; snow alone, ice, mud, and binding blankets with static electricity will affect your horse's healing. Blankets will greatly limit their already-limited mobility, but are necessary to keep them warm. The cold makes a horse much more reactive to his environment and excited at work or walk time.

Getting yourself to and from the indoor arena must be planned if your barn is not connected to the arena. Ice, snow, and mud can be a disastrous condition, especially if you only have an outdoor arena. Any soft-tissue leg injury must be protected at this time, and these environmental challenges can have serious potential complications. There are many rehabilitation barns in warmer climates that you may need to consider as an option, even if it is for only the toughest parts of the seasons. If you have to ship your horse to a rehabilitation facility, be careful not to have a steep trailer ramp. He must be monitored carefully on any trip; he is not fit, and is quite weak. The trip will be exhausting for him and this must be recognized as a potential complication. Discuss with your veterinarian supportive methods of shipment, fluids, medications, and an altered travel plan. This may include multiple stays at veterinary clinics on the way to your destination.

There are many rehabilitation clinics around the country. Some are extensions of veterinary clinics and some are privately owned; these clinics focus primarily on reconditioning and rehabilitating horses. They should have well-trained staff members who are familiar with all aspects of rehabilitation. Some of these facilities work with veterinary schools and clinics, and have access to many wonderful rehabilitation machines, treadmills, and advanced modalities that can help with the healing process. This may get costly, so be prepared to utilize the time when you may really need it the most. Please recognize that this is not the miracle answer for 100 percent soundness either; these are trained people who will do the best they can for your horse. The Internet can also provide vital information and avenues of support.

FOOD FOR THOUGHT

If your injury occurs or is managed at the time of year when it is cold, this part of rehabilitation starts to get a bit tricky; you do not want to overfeed your horse to make up for the calories he needs to heal. And you must cut his grain intake back because he is not working under normal conditions. All the omega fats are essential for normal body functions. Horses utilize fat for stored energy; this also allows us to feed the horse much less in grain rations. The omega fats are also helpful in reducing inflammation in the horse's body. Here is where you need to do some feeding homework. There are resources online, and some that veterinary schools offer. I had great feedback from a Dr. Deb Valentine at Oregon

State University. She is a pathologist who has done extensive work on fat in the equine diet. Her studies focus mainly on equine polysaccharide myopathy (EPSM), but her work is also informative as to the nutritional demands of equines. She is a wonderful contact for fat supplementation in an equine diet. Feed companies, universities, and colleges may be able to help develop a plan for your injured horse's feed program. You can easily contact these facilities either by e-mail or phone; they have educated nutritionists willing and available for you to question.

You will need to give your horse some grain product to help support the body during the healing process, but at some point in this process, the horse will possibly look a bit skinny and unfit. Many times during the rehabilitation process, the horse will lose significant weight. This will help to have less weight for the horse to carry as he is rehabilitating. But as they start to heal and need to get strong for the active part of their working program, the feed program must be dynamic and change, as will the needs of the horse. A higher-fat- more fiber based diet may be a better choice during this time. The fat will give the horse a "cool energy," and allow you to feed a much smaller portion and still provide nutritional requirements. The lower the protein in the feeds, the better at this point in the healing process, we do not need the extra energy. The horse's feed program must keep changing as do the horse's needs; the seasonal changes must be considered in the program as well. The seasons have a significant role in rehabilitation, as to the demands they have on the horse's natural body. Horses are photosensitive, they shed their hair according to the seasons, and they have a spring shed for their summer coat, a fall shed for their winter coat and a winter shed for their spring coat. There are significant metabolic changed that are naturally occurring during this seasonal time change. This absolutely needs to be taken under consideration for all horses, much less a rehabilitating horse.

Make sure you can offer good-quality hay for your horse; he does not need any alfalfa or high-energy food at this time. Hay cubes may be a good idea; they require the horse to take time to eat, use energy, and pace their feed time. Hay cubes are not good for horses that eat fast; this could lead to choking. A good-quality grass hay or timothy is sufficient. I highly recommend wetting the hay, especially since the horses are stuck inside so much. This will help get the dust out of the hay, and also gives the horse more fluid intake. I always try to keep some hay in front of my horses at all times, even if it is a flake every couple of hours. Wetting a large amount of hay can sometimes get smelly, and he will not eat it. Try not to let him have long periods of time without any food. If possible, a very good practice to get into with all stall-kept horse programs is to provide some nighttime hay as well, a few flakes between eight and ten o'clock at night is ideal. Horses were created to graze constantly; acids will build up in their stomachs, and stress comes into their lives from no turnout and minimum work. When the horse grazes he produces buffers in his saliva that neutralize the acids in his stomach, therefore preventing over stimulation of acid production in the stomach. If a horse is not initially provided at feeding time a grazing, grass or hay type product and only fed first a high grain based diet he becomes very susceptible to gastrointestinal issues. Hay cubes should be a possibility in areas that do not have access to hay. One should **never** feed grain to horses that have an empty stomach, and never ride a horse on an empty stomach. The acid production in a horse is amazing and destructive. It will lead to ulcers and other gastrointestinal problems that could potentionaly arise as behavioral issues. Keep this in mind for your program!

Supplement Suggestions

Vitamin E, selenium, and zinc support soft-tissue cell repair. You will need to keep your horse on some kind of supplement. Selenium needs to be handled with care, as selenium poisoning can occur if the soil levels test high in the hay and grass the horse is consuming. This is dependent on the area in which one lives. Hay and grass samples can be sent to the USDA to be tested for their selenium values, as well as other nutritional values. Vitamin C is great to support the immune system. A complete mineral and vitamin supplement of some type will support the healing process. There are also supplements on the market designed specifically for these cases. Read your ingredients so you do not waste your money and feed too much of the same supplement! You may need to remember to include a calming supplement or even gastrointestinal support. The omega fats are essential in an equine diet, regardless of an injury. There is a great deal of information available on how they help decrease inflammation and aid in tissue repair from many resources, one must investigate these areas, I cannot give assistance to my readers as I am only accounting for my experiences. Joint supplementation is crucial as well. Feed supplements can include: MSM as an anti-inflammatory, hyluronic acid for proper joint function, and glucosamine as well. There are supplements your vet can also provide as a medicinal course of injections, such as Adequan and Legend for joint support and function.

Do not think that taking your horse off his supplements at this crucial time is a good idea; he needs them and will benefit from nutritional support as well.

CHAPTER ELEVEN
Proprioception: Knowing Where to Put Your Feet

As defined by me: the ability of the restricted, rehabilitating horse to be in any unfamiliar and unstable tangible environment due to his limb-related limitations or incidents due to an injury or illness. Simply put: The horse will lose his perception to move normally within his environment when he is restricted to his stall. He will trip, get wobbly in his gait, and become uncoordinated when he moves.

I have personally discovered that the horse that is able to go without wearing shoes during this time is quicker to regain his Proprioception than the horse that has shoes on. In some horses, this will not be possible, due to the conditions of their hooves, the environment, and possible support issues shoeing may provide. This is also true of the horse that is able to be taken out of the stall more frequently. Age is a factor of consideration; the younger horse ideally will have a quicker and better success rate. History of the horse is important at this point, as is exposure to being in multiple environments versus a consistent environment. A facility that provides a consistent footing surface is ideal in the beginning phases of a rest-and-rehabilitation program; the harder the surface the better. Gradual challenges should be included only after a canter program has been established for a minimum of three months. These challenges may include small-incline hills, mud and backing exercises, smaller-type circles, lateral work, and uneven footing. Footing considerations need to be noted for the rest of the horse's life.

CHAPTER TWELVE
Alternative Therapies
THE FEEL-GOOD STUFF! MASSAGE, ACUPUNCTURE, CHIROPRACTOR, CRANIAL SACRAL WORK, AND MYOFACIAL RELEASE TECHNIQUES

Spend your money wisely during this time

Whether you believe or not ... try some of these techniques on yourself first. If you are a non-believer, the best proof of unfamiliar experiences is to have one of your own!

On your road to recovery, you have juvenile healing tissue and things are going pretty well. We have worked out many of the ugly details of rest, and are now facing the months of consistent therapies. Rehabilitation now becomes the issue of time. As this time passes, education must happen. Your horse's fitness is rapidly diminishing, he is very limited in his movement, and his body is weak. He also is not healed. So, like us, when a part of our body aches, we use other means to compensate for the weakness of the larger stabilizing muscles. But one must recognize that those smaller compensatory muscles are weak as well, and doing twice their original job. They are making up for the larger damaged tendons and ligaments. So let us keep yet another dynamic in mind!

You need to remember to address the horse's entire body, not solely the injury. This will play a major part in bringing the horse's fitness level back when he can start to work. I recommend using massage, myofacial release, chiropractic, and acupuncture as part of an entire process of healing. It can get very expensive, but the benefits are worth the cost. Remember, you cannot go to any horse shows for at least six months, so spend your money on therapies. Letting another professional put his hands on your horse helps give you, the owner/rider, a better perspective of the healing process. Your eyes are looking at the same horse every day. Let a fresh pair of eyes help you see any problems that will arise. As always, the more one can do with these therapies the better. So in any scenario, trying to get at least one of these practices routinely involved in your program will assist the entire horse.

The professional alternative manual healers will also give you ideas and exercises that you can practice on a daily basis. With these natural healing arts, find the best. A good healer will take a good period of time to assess and work on your horse. A twenty-minute "dust and fluff" massage is not enough. Find a well-educated and experienced certified equine massage therapist. The good ones should be certified; you can ask them if they are and check out their credentials. If you are using any healer who does not find the same issues that you are feeling in your horse, that person may be not the best to use at this time. Be true to yourself as well, and remember you know your horse and must be comfortable with whomever you work with. I must say, be careful as well; equine enthusiasts can become emotionally sensitive during this time and can fall victim to those who have limited professional knowledge but are telling vulnerable people what they need and want to hear. They will gladly listen to your story and your issues for a price! Be cautious here.

I find it best to combine therapies; there are many different methods of chiropractic and acupuncture therapy. These therapies should be performed by veterinarians, and if they are not veterinarians, then a discussion and the support of your veterinarian must be included. The practitioner must be qualified. Some veterinarians are so successful with methods of treatment, they actually focus primarily on therapies. I mention this only to help you use your money wisely, and not waste your money on false practitioners.

Notice how his left shoulder is higher than his right and the left hip is higher than the right.

Visual information

Please note the asymmetry in Buddy's right and left shoulders, as well as the difference in the hip height of the diagonal pair. This is quite common. The horse "postures" when he has an injured limb, which means in lay terms that the horse tends not to put weight on the painful limb, and compensates with the other limbs. Standing off the injured leg produces an asymmetry, muscle atrophy, and over-development on the strong side. This is a pictorial example of the need for multiple professional inputs. This is a more dramatic picture of asymmetry because there are also other physiological factors involved with this particular horse.

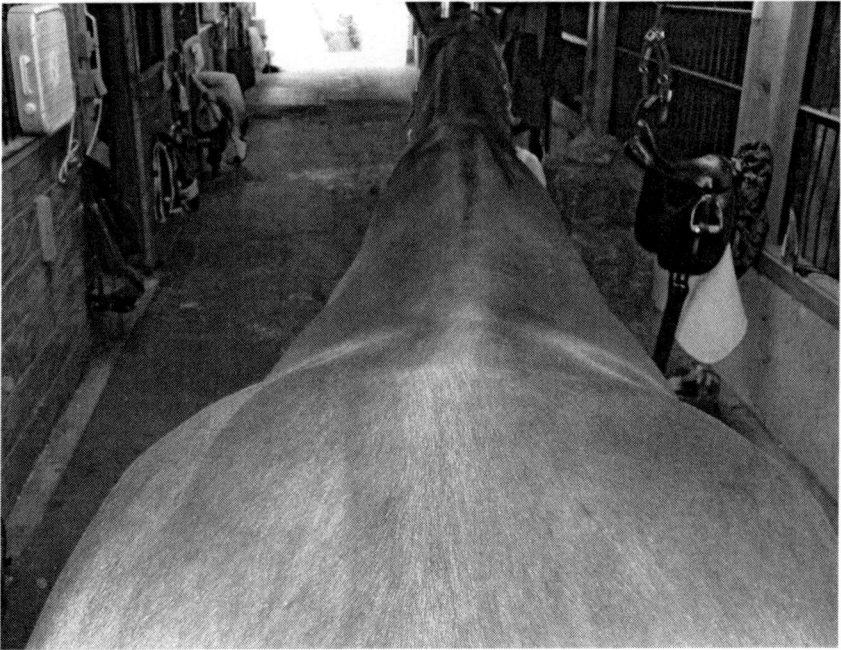

Muscle atrophy of left shoulder and twist in pelvis

Chapter Thirteen
NOTE: *Symmetry and Shoeing*

I will briefly give my reader some basic information on shoeing; this area has been a highly discussed topic for many years but I will give a few basic tidbits of information that should be a constant.

Firstly, put the horse on cross-ties, and get something you can stand on without scaring the horse. Get on a milk crate or something solid, so that you can look from behind him, down his back, up his neck and to his head and see what the spine looks like. Your horse must stand fairly square when you are doing this, is his spine straight? Is one side higher than the other? Look at the shoulders and hips; compare the left and right sides. Then look at the knees and hocks as well. Are they level? This is invaluable information; if the horse is not balanced, level, or even on both sides of his body from the *ground level*, he will be compensatory and develop uneven musculature, multiple body issues and potential future lameness. Some degree of asymmetry is acceptable and normal for horses, but anything extreme must be noted as areas of concern. Other causes of muscular asymmetry can be managed by a qualified chiropractor and massage therapist.

Secondly, when the horse walks, his hooves must hit the ground level or flat. The horse must first be balanced from the ground, or his feet. The horse must break over his shoe or hoof in the middle of his shoe or hoof.

This means when you look at the shoe off the hoof or look at the horse's hoof, he must have wear marks in the middle of the hoof. If the break over wear mark is not in the middle of the hoof or shoe, the horse is not balanced. The hoof should not roll when it lands on the ground to the outside or inside of the hoof. You can use the angle of the shoulder and the angle of the stifle to the hip as a reference point. These angles must be the same as the angles of the pastern bones; that is they should be the same angle as the bones of the foot are in the hoof capsule. That is the natural boney alignment of each particular horse and each particular leg. This is invaluable knowledge; angles and discussions of them are useless if the horse is not sound. A crooked-leg horse is just that; "fixing" the mature horse's crooked leg will be his demise. Supporting a crooked-leg horse could be considered a soundness miracle to some. As always, there are a few of those horses that make us all just have to accept—that is the way they are and they break all the rules in the books. They make all of our education seem useless, these are the horses we just scratch our heads and go HMM? How does that horse move with those legs and feet and stay sound?

Horses that have toes that are too long usually are "trippy." Forging or horses that interfere can be a bit more complicated. That is a balance issue that involves both the rider and the farrier working together to prob-lem-solve. If the farrier cuts off too much heel from the horse, and the fur of the horse's heel bulbs touches the ground, this puts an enormous amount of strain on the tendons of the leg. Also, by not balancing a horse that has a flat foot and a high hoof—commonly known as a club-footed horse—is a mistake. This I have experienced to be an excuse for many persons' reasons as to why their horse is not sound, but this shoeing issue has a solution when you and your farrier work together. Balance starts from the ground level and the foundation of the horse must be level and balanced. It is your farrier's responsibility to make this not be part of the lameness equation. The rest becomes another world of equine issues and areas of discovery!

You build a house from a foundation, not the attic.

Chapter Fourteen
Therapeutic Modalities
Lasers

It is my experience that lasers have helped assist with the healing process. Ligaments and tendons take a very long time to heal. Why? Because the blood and oxygen supplies to these areas are not very efficient. Blood and oxygen restore damaged tissue and regenerate healthy tissue. The slower the blood supply, the longer the healing time. Think in terms of your own body. Recall how quickly your mouth heals after a trip to the dentist, and how much you bleed when you cut your lip. The closer the blood is to the surface, the more you bleed, and the quicker you heal.

Now let's recognize where the horse's heart is: up high in the middle of his mass. Let us acknowledge how little muscle mass is in the lower leg, and how much energy it takes to send the blood down to the limb and then pump it all the way back up the leg and then back to the heart! That is quite a long trip under normal circumstances, let alone in the case of an injury that demands even more attention. What the laser does is help stimulate the blood flow to the area of injury. Inflammation slows down the flow of blood, so getting the inflammation out and getting more blood in is of major importance. The laser seems to be very effective for assisting this.

There are different types of lasers; they can be expensive if purchased, but some veterinary clinics rent them, or you can get treatments by a qualified technician. You must learn about how to use this equipment properly if you are able to purchase one. It is necessary to understand the safety issues, for yourself and the horse, when you use a laser. You must wear protective glasses and not leave the laser on the injured tissue more than the recommended time. You can damage the tissue if you do not understand how to use this therapy. Most people will have a difficult time buying one for therapeutic reasons, unless a veterinarian approves one for you. The protocols and procedures for the use of lasers will be documented by the companies.

Chi Machines: This is a very user-friendly, safe machine, and not as expensive as a laser, but it has been my experience that this technique does seem to give the horses great benefits. This form of therapy uses a type of sound waves to move blocked energy within the body and allow the energy to be released. Energy gets blocked when a system does not operate properly—a basic clog in the pipe. In this case, we are relating to the horse's energy and the damage his leg has sustained. So it unblocks areas that get locked or tired, or are ill. The horses really seem to enjoy this machine, too. It is also useful for many other conditions. Web sites can offer more info as to success. It is a more of a natural medicine approach, and quite a bit safer for an inexperienced horseperson to use.

Shockwave Therapy: Shockwave therapy is in the same vein as the above, but is done under the guidance of a veterinarian and is much more sophisticated. Shockwave therapy utilizes high-energy acoustic pulses like sound waves. These waves have the ability to travel through soft tissue, and seem to reduce the response of the mechanisms that cause pain in the body. This therapy assists the break-up of the scar tissue that can interfere with proper healing tissue alignment. The horse usually requires sedation for this procedure because the levels of "pulses" that are needed are quite intense and literally feel like an electrical shock. This therapy can be expensive and should be performed a minimum of three times for any beneficial results.

SURGICAL PROCEDURES:

When a horse has an injury that does not respond to the conventional treatments of "normal" rehabilitation, there will be some horses that require a surgical procedure as an option.

Again, cost may be an issue, as well as future usefulness. All veterinary procedures and information should be explained in depth by your veterinarian prior to this event. The possible mobility limitations and risks involved in any surgical procedures, as well as the costs, will become necessary information at this time. Surgical procedures can make a significant difference in the horse's usefulness and healing response. There are many surgeons who are also combining the PRP procedure with the surgeries and having very good results. Some traumatic injuries may not have another option, and surgical procedures will be necessary. Also, with any of these areas, utilize a veterinary surgeon who specializes in these types of surgeries.

Use what you can and trash what you cannot use. —R.K.

Stem Cell Therapy: This area, for some, may be ethically controversial, but the information has value. Stem cells are immature cells produced by the body and used to replace tissue damage in any form. Stem cell therapy involves harvesting stem cells, normally from the horse to be treated. The cells are taken from either bone marrow or adipose (fat tissue). The tissue is sent to a specialized facility and multiplied by cell culture. The purified cell sample is then transported back to the veterinarian, who then injects it into the injury site. The stem cells produce new tissue to replace the damaged tendon tissue. There are risks, as with any procedure, of infection and other complications. This is also an expensive procedure but usually only requires a one-time injection. All this, as I keep reminding my readers, must be discussed with your veterinarian.

Plasma-rich Protein: This procedure involves usage of a syringe to take a sample of blood out of the horse's body, use of a centrifuge to spin the blood down, separating the horse's blood and extracting the plasma. The plasma has qualities that can assimilate into any injured area they are injected into. This is a fantastic advance in soft-tissue healing; there is little chance of rejection, because the blood is taken from the same host. A more advanced method of therapy and a costly one, but if the success rate is better, the cost is worth the investment. I have recently read of this procedure in human injuries as well.

Comment: *Both stem cell and PRP are fantastic options, and recently, many documented studies support these options. As of now, there are veterinary facilities that are actually committed to both of these therapies.*

Chapter Fifteen
Walking and Eventual Trot-like Exercises

When you can have a walk program, make the best of your time. You have established a work ethic for your horse, right? Now he can use it in the walk. Be smart about this; make sure you have hand-walked or grazed your horse and gotten the dangerous energy out of him before you get on him. I recommend at least twenty minutes of hand-walk or hand-graze before you get on. But, **I *must also state*** that some horses are better off to be in their tack and working first and hand-grazed after work; some horses were impossible to hand-graze and only would work. I have had young horses that, by putting on the saddle and the bridle, were much better to handle simply because they were in their "work clothes." So, assessments of age and training are also a variable to be considered.

Now let us take the reins and move. This is not a trail ride. Have a solid hold on the reins, but do not trap the horse; let him walk, marching forward, under control. If you make the reins too tight and make the horse's neck too short, the horse will get nervous and panicky. Horses are flight-or-fight animals. Let him have a bit of the flight instinct. Use this as your area of focus. Fight is definitely the other instinct you do not want to reveal, and keeping the reins too tight can bring this response out.

The horse needs to maintain a flat-footed, clear, four-beat walk rhythm. If the horse's neck gets too short and tight when you walk, you run the risk of making him get lateral or pacing at the walk gait. This is a very difficult fault to correct. So, allow the horse to have his neck and make him march in the walk gait.

NEXT: Do not assume the horse will be in the same mindset every day.

A nice long walk will be the best thing for healing and conditioning— a free walk with a controlled long rein, **always under control.** Utilize your voice commands: Halt … Walk … Halt … not pressure or training, just busy work: forty-five minutes once or twice a day for the horse's working mind. Consult your veterinarian, and discuss your exercise plan. These are my ideas, and again, every situation is unique. This is the recommendation for the classic injury, not a traumatic injury, and may help the reader understand the ultimate goal.

This idea should only be used with a front-leg injury, not a hind-leg injury:

This idea may be a possibility after at least an extended walk program at the minimum of five months is established, without any changes to the leg, and only executed by an advanced horse and rider. If you have an extremely well-trained and advanced horse, utilize your "kind" dressage piaffe work. If you have a much less advanced horse, the idea is controlled movement. You must be able to make your horse take three steps of trot and walk as if it is not a big deal. The injured horse can easily work with very little momentum. It is mentally and physically exhausting for the horse, and is a good physical therapy exercise. The exercises of the piaffe—technically known to dressage riders as "half-steps"—requires a very simple work idea: lift your leg and put it down. Once the horse has walked for at least thirty minutes, use five non-consecutive minutes of piaffe-like steps or trot-like steps to strengthen, challenge, and therapeutically stretch the tendons. This work also helps the horse's mind get tired. This idea, by all means, does not require on-the-spot performance piaffe, merely letting the educated horse work his advanced mind a bit. He must have **many** rest breaks, and work always on a fairly loose rein;

he also must not do this on the daily rehabilitation work. I would utilize my long-line techniques with a well-behaved horse. I would sometimes prefer to utilize the long lines during this time; they involve no carrying weight and simple movements that I can control and slowly develop, I can also watch for any soundness changes. It is the *idea* of the piaffe movements you are utilizing, not the demands. It could be equated to a person with a minor knee injury. After you are able to walk and the rest period of your therapy is finished, the therapist may put you on a stationary bike to create a different therapeutic movement. He doesn't expect you to do the Tour de France.

Again, I must remind my readers, I am a professional dressage trainer and these are merely my concepts and program ideas that worked well for me. They may not be possible for all of the folks who read my manual.

The horse will get tired in a good way, and you will always remain in control. I discovered that initially, the horse needs to get back into shape after his rest period, so your actual riding program is greatly altered and enhanced by this work. When I would do my trot-like work, I would only work for forty-five minutes, versus a walk-only program of an hour. I would always change my time spent on the horse when I added to my program, because a new concept is a new demand, and that alone on the recovering horse is a challenge.

Next: Getting ready to do some work

The ultrasound looks good, and our injured tissue is healed. This has been six months for many, and a very long time.

Now that we have been given the green light to start to do any type of work with the horse, we must realize that now begins the process that all of your religious discipline has been preparing you for. Remember, your horse is very weak. He may still be leaping and rearing in his stall, but all his muscles have some degree of atrophy. If you have not been able to walk your horse under tack, this can get very dangerous.

I still recommend keeping to your program, walking him in hand first, just like you have been doing. Let the horse have a graze for forty-five minutes, if you have the time prior to your riding time and if grass is available. If grass is not available, then a hand walk is still an option prior to the riding part of his program. Remember as well, some horses will do better to be worked prior to being hand-grazed. You must know your horse! If one is not able to hand-graze, then be highly disciplined in your exercise program and be very unemotional and businesslike in your management time.

Every horse is different during his program and when it is time to work. Some will be fine; some will be wild. But above all, be safe. Put on a set of draw reins, assuming you know how to use them. Use of the double bridle—for those who can—may be the option. Use some piece of equipment or training device that will give you control and a safe rehabilitation. A more serious bit may be necessary for this interim. You are not "training" your horse, you are avoiding getting hurt, and your goal is to stay on and safely work your horse. Your training will stay there and be there when you get to train again. If you feel your training will suffer because you insist on using a gentle bit on your thousand-pound, pent-up, ready-to-explode, stuck-in-the-stall-for-six-months crazy beast, you need to re-assess your skills as a trainer. As an amateur, do not use your emotional thought process, utilize your practical knowledge. Be careful and wear your helmet. Most horses get very happy when they can trot. Mine have given me squeals just by shortening the reins. They get a hump in their back, and have impressed me with their "rehabilitation" buck. The horse does not know that he will only make five trot steps and that's it. So he needs to stop after these steps. Make him stop. He will learn what steps are. He will even count with you.

When you have built your exercise program and can trot, your vet will need to give you recommendations for how much you can actually do. I will share my ideas. Ask your vet his opinion. I have a conservative program that some may find too slow.

The Ideal Riding and Rehabilitation Program Starts with a Good Ultrasound Scan

My Program:

No lunging of the horse at all!

No small—less than twenty-meter—circles.

No collection for the dressage horses.

If the horse can ground drive or longe line, one can utilize this in the rehabilitation program, remembering the same restrictions, and be aware of the challenges. This is an advanced concept and we do not want the long lines getting tangled in our newly healed leg!

You must have connected rein contact when you can ride them, do not allow the horse to run on the forehand and drag you around the work arena; you will discover his comfort level of work as the rider. The horse will feel as if he has four square wheels as legs when you begin to walk and trot; do not be confused by this. It will be necessary to work through this uneven, uncomfortable gait, provided the injured leg displays no changes of heat or swelling.

Insist on a controlled marching walk rhythm and controlled rein length.

Hard surface is a **must,** with flat, solid footing. No soft, deep, uneven, or slippery footing. A careful consideration of mud and sand, during the off seasons, must be a constant appreciation when one is rehabilitating the horse. A safe environment may be a consideration as well; a contained and enclosed area.

Straight lines only; minimal arc circles at the most should be used. Small, bending circles create unnecessary stress on the leg at this healing point.

Assuming that you have been able to keep an activity level in your grade one or grade two lame injured horse, your progress after a six month rest and walk-only program may begin as this program and only after a clean ultrasound:

Week 1: Walk 20 minutes, trot 5 steps, possibly 10.

Week 2: Walk 20 minutes, trot 10 steps.

Week 3: Walk 20 minutes, trot 20 steps.

Week 4: Walk 20 minutes, trot 30 steps.

Week 5: Same; add 10 trot steps each week.

Week 9: Same; add trot steps until 5 minutes of trot are solid.

Remember to take breaks; total work time and trot steps can be met with frequent walk breaks. Always take the time to warm up and cool down properly, twenty minutes of walk work can be in the arena, but the horse can walk or hack in solid footing for a longer period of time before and after his "work" program.

This I recommend for the first month and a half during your "back to work" time.

During this work time, you must be aware of how your horse is healing. If the horse displays any signs of any heat, lameness, or swelling anywhere in his body, particularly at the site of injury, this program needs to change **immediately** to accommodate the horse. You must notify your veterinarian if any of these changes happen. There is some remodeling of the tissue that will cause changes to the leg and can cause heat and swelling. You must treat this the same way you did when the injury started: poultice, anti-inflamatories, and rest, again.

During the second month of rehabilitation exercise, you should be able to turn the trot steps into minutes, building the horse's rehabilitation trot program weekly in five-minute increments. Again, remember to keep assessing your horse's healing process. You may note a little puffiness around the injury site when you start to trot; this is common. This swelling should go down after the horse moves. If it does not, consult your vet. The injury site is continuing to remodel, and the collagen fibers require exercise to heal and align properly, reducing scar tissue, of the healed tissue that has fluid, blood, and scar tissue in it at this point; these are issues you will need to work through. Unfortunately, this is part of the rehabilitation process. Understanding the entire program is vital to a successful recovery. We are trying to avoid having this "puffiness" of the injury become a permanent blemish. Reducing the scar tissue and controlling the healing process is our ultimate goal; to get 100 percent of healing and minimal scar tissue is optimal.

RE-ULTRASOUND BEFORE YOU CANTER

Utilize very large circles over twenty meters
Week 1: Walk 20 minutes, trot 10 minutes, canter 5 minutes.

Week 2: Walk 20 minutes, trot 15 minutes, canter 10 minutes.
Week 3: Walk 20 minutes, trot 20 minutes, canter 20 minutes.

Remember that these sessions must be **total** work times, **not consecutive work times.** The time reference is only to help with the total rehabilitation program. This work time has now become months of rehabilitation and work. What was "normal" before will be forever changed. Assessments must be considered forever for your injured horse. This injury will be healed and resolved, but should always remain in your thoughts. It is never "over"; do not pretend in your mind that everything is back to normal. Your horse and you went through a very long process, and you must continue to respect that time.

If you have a more advanced dressage horse, you can continue to use the "*idea*" of piaffe for strength and mental challenge. Just the simple idea of lifting his feet is enough of a demand on those ligaments and muscles. If you have a well-trained horse and can do five steps of simple forward trot, and use the movement as a therapeutic exercise, this is a great addition to your program. Again, one must remember to have a constant discussion of any program with your veterinarian.

I suggest following this program for two more weeks before starting any forms of lateral work and small jumping fences. You still cannot lunge your horse and not let him experience hills, muddy trails, sandy beaches, deep sand, and no steep trailer ramps if you need to move him.

As the rider doing the physical therapy on your horse, you need to keep remembering that your once-familiar, wonderful-feeling horse is going to feel awful when you start to move. He will feel stiff, tight, resistant, and heavy in the bridle, and may pull on your hands. He will also be crooked and have many other awful feelings. Do not despair; he is moving. **Remember where you came from.** He was standing in his stall and only walking six months ago. This is a very hard time to acknowledge … again, but we are now looking at the eighth month of our program and a sound horse due to your educated hard work.

You are just getting the horse into moving, and fitness is the task. It is not fair to you or your horse to assume that he can collect himself, get up, and go. He cannot do it; he is terribly weak, so focus on fitness. Let him be a little flat, connected so he is under control, but not feeling the way he feels before you go into the show ring. This will take time. How much? Each horse and rider is different. Remember that there is significant muscle atrophy. The horse's top-line muscles will go away; your saddle will not fit your horse properly, and may need to be altered, and other issues may arise as the horse's body has changed during this dynamic time.

He will start to get slowly stronger. You also need to adjust his diet as he becomes fitter. Slowly increase his food, so you can start helping him regain lost muscle. About every two weeks, after you are trotting for twenty minutes, you will notice many changes. Your horse usually begins to feel more normal. Your riding time will start off better and better. You must realize that the horse will quickly tire. So be conscious of this time; use the starting time as a reference. The longer he feels good, the stronger he is getting, and the more you can give him to eat. It becomes a very tricky balance. You need to feed him to get him strong and feel more like you remembered him. There are a series of constant dynamic events that come from these injuries. Remember to keep attention to the leg and notice any changes that could possibly occur. These events were my motivations for writing my experiences down, and hopefully I have given some insight as to the depth of this time.

The injured horse may have to face a different lifestyle and never be able to have turnout or lunge again. This is dependent on the injury, environment, and horse. Every time you go anywhere, you must be aware of the footing! Seriously consider, for the years after the injury, that you can challenge this injury constantly and have implications. Personally, I am obsessive about the surface my horse works on, competes on, gets turned out on, and trail rides on. It is necessary information to have in the back of your mind forever. For those of you who are event riders or jumpers or any other performance rider, I offer just a little food for thought on future practices.

Really take the time to re-assess your conditions and slowly introduce the horse back to any new type of footing. Building him up gradually to his conditions, remember that his injured leg is not the same as it was, and it never will be again.

CHAPTER SIXTEEN
Turnout

***After your horse is healed, it will take at the minimum of double
his down time to get him back to work.***

You may be able to reintroduce your regular, normal riding equipment at
this time. But each day, as we must remember, is not like the one before.
So approach none of the days assuming the "same old thing." Some injuries
will require a much longer timeframe. This is only my template for you to
use and modify. But don't think cutting corners and starting earlier is a
smart decision; it will cost you threefold in the long run. You have already
lost a year of showing, and committed to this program; use your time and
knowledge for a healthy future for your friend.

I do not recommend any turnout of your horse out until he is canter-
ing at a minimum for the first month and there are no noticeable changes
in the injury. Because, as you have experienced at this point of your horse's
rehabilitation, your horse will only want to go out into a paddock and
run, buck, and get crazy, when allowed to be turned out after this time
uncontrolled. So you need to remember that you are potentially getting
him reconditioned for any type of a turnout time and normal usefulness.
It is your responsibility to prevent him from hurting himself again. After
all this time, you really don't want to lose all your rehabilitation work. I

have found that if I can stick with this routine for six months, incorporate the ride, and then do a short, supervised turnout, the ultimate goal would be a safe, normal turnout program again.

Be systematic, when you do decide you want to turn him out. Take a bucket of grain, treats, or carrots, and leave it near the gate. Turn him out at a quiet time, alone or near a quiet horse, and in a **small paddock** or round pen—nothing larger than twenty meters—to prevent him from going too fast. Stay with him in the paddock when you decide to wean the horse of your constant connection, to YOU.

I start this time as a hand-graze, after our work time. This has been a familiar routine in his life this far. If you do not have grass, put some hay out for him to graze on. I would then carefully unsnap the horse from the lunge line, very slowly and without event. I would stay with him, and pick the rocks out of the field, and the manure or weeds. Fifteen to thirty minutes is long enough. If it goes well, then continue this program daily, a bit longer each time, but keep in mind that your horse is not used to being left alone, and a full-day turnout only exhausts him at this time, and can lead to a longer recovery and recurrent injury. When I was able to wean my horse from the lunge line, I would take a chair, a bucket of grain, and a book, and "baby-sit" the horse for an hour before I even considered leaving him alone. It took a good six months before I ever left him out longer than an hour.

Do not give up; you are at a very critical place.

I have heard too many sad stories of others who have had to rehabilitate their horse from a soft-tissue leg injury.

I have heard **too** many people tell me, "My vet said I could turn my horse out. "He ran around like crazy, in his (old) paddock," [which no one knows the size of but you!] "Now he is lame again."

After six months of rest and rehabilitation work, this is an unfortunate and preventable mistake. This is avoidable, because a specific program was not discussed as to the work and turnout program; this is an extremely important time and must be regarded as such.

On top of that, the horse has probably pulled every muscle in his very weak, stall-bound body.

Horse owners have told me:

"I could not bear to see my horse so depressed when his friends were playing in the field."

A horse will adjust. Do not put your human emotions on him; just understand his **SITUATION.** Your sole purpose for rehabilitation is to get your horse back, fit for turnout and riding. Let us always keep this in mind. It will be hard enough to prevent him from hurting himself when you are handling him, and to just unleash him after all this time you have invested … it's not the way to go. Your risk of re-injuries and multiple injuries would triple, as would your timeframe.

So don't turn your horse out until he is fit again. Please!

Over a period of time, I could detach myself and re-educate my horse to be able to live a normal turned-out life. Again, I repeat myself, but this has been a long journey and some topics must be heard again.

As we must part

I am near the end of my manual; I hope I have given my readers some useful and helpful information. I cannot provide you information as to what may happen, what could happen, what will or will not happen, and what has happened; I can only provide information at this point of my experience as to what I have gathered to write my manual. I wish you the best of luck and health.

Buddy and Me

I cannot properly express the gratitude I have for all the people who supported and helped me through this very trying time—my husband (I am so fortunate to have found a man like Eric), my family, and friends. All of my professional friends were great sources of knowledge through this eternity, and offered ideas and words of encouragement. My veterinarian, Dr. John Lockamy, was the most phenomenal veterinarian any person could have to help guide them through this journey. And it was through discovery, reading, and gaining knowledge through experienced professionals that I was able to share with you my story of rehabilitation. Good information and wrong information as well have been my insight.

I have personally been through three equine injuries—or just really bad luck. One injury was a trailer accident. Buddy somehow got his right foreleg entangled in his hay net on the way to a horse show. Did I hang the net too low, the same way I always had hung it? Did I make a mistake somewhere? I can tell you that I use a hay bag now and will never put a hay net up again!

It was just an unfortunate accident. He hurt his check ligament and this resulted in one year of recovery.

The second injury I know was work-related. I changed my training program. I knew better, but … that's another story. Oddly enough, though the injury was to the digital flexor tendon, it is my belief that it started from his back, shoulder, and neck becoming overworked. We were training to be candidates for the Pan American Games and be a potential Grand Prix dressage competitor, but by riding too much passage—as advised by a well-known dressage trainer—Buddy then exhausted his back, neck, and shoulder muscles. I thought I could ride him through the tight back problem instead of resting him; I pushed and he finally strained the flexor ligament. To this day, I question any trainer who requires a horse to work repetitively in the passage to develop strength for the Grand Prix. A combined total program develops strength through fitness, not repetitive motion. Ten months' recovery time on a fourteen-year-old horse is a turning point in both of our lives, and means many, many setbacks. Buddy has a lovely piaffe and passage, and easily gives these *"gifts of movement" to his rider.* A huge fault of the sport I am in is the lack of knowledge professionals have as to the training scale and the developmental processes of upper-level movements. That was my two-second soapbox speech. Buddy is a fourth-level horse that has all the Grand Prix movements; he gets too tense during the tests to perform competitively. His tension could be from his injuries and performance pressure he feels. I must take this into account, for him and myself, and that is okay. We have shown in New England and Florida, where we live. He is now nineteen years old and has given me so much as my friend, travel companion, competition partner, and teacher. I am very blessed to have been able to have learned so much from him. He was a difficult horse to train, and most of my work was done alone. We have had a few select persons who have helped us, and we were very fortunate to have found those who were true horsemen and not opportunists.

My third horse injury was my young Grand Prix prospect horse, Elvis. A reckless accident; a negligent maintenance worker on a lawn mower scared Elvis, and he fell down hard on his left side. He injured the meniscus of his stifle and tore his hind limb suspensory ligament at the point of attachment. Elvis was a surgical candidate and was misdiagnosed for more than a year; "this mistake" has extended his rehabilitation into a two-year project. His future is undetermined at his point.

I am not rich; I do not have a trainer on call or another horse to continue on at this time. All of our successes and all of our failures are mine. But hard work, many miles of mistakes, and the sacrifice of many hard-earned dollars—included with the emotions of striving to reach a monumental personal goal—were my motivations to help others.

I still believe very strongly in classical training, and it is a shame that true classical training is disappearing in the sport of dressage. The training of the horse should be all-encompassing. There should be limited and reasonable excuses for "why the horse can't" do something versus what he can do. To wear a Shadbelly when I discovered dressage was an honor of accomplishment; now it is about buying the horse that can make you look good, wearing the right clothes, and displaying a false status. It is no longer a merit of a true classical accomplishment. It is very sad to me that so many have sold out for superficial gain, when true accomplishments are so much more affordable and satisfying.

I have had some amazing guidance by some very special trainers. Those of you know who you are, and I cannot thank you enough for your knowledge and help. My future horses will receive the gifts of knowledge from Buddy, and open new doors for us. Buddy will continue to work for all his days; he will always have a job. But I retired him from serious competition after the last injury. I want a healthy, sound horse much more than the cost of a $1,500 horse-show weekend and a forty-cent blue ribbon.

I have shown him in lower levels after his injuries; he is fine now, but I value our relationship too much. Who he is and what he means to me supersedes my goals. Enough is enough. I guess the last injury I relate to my greediness to succeed. It cost me way too much emotionally and almost destroyed my partner. I know so much more now to trust myself and know I am a knowledgeable trainer and horseman. No one, no matter how many ribbons he has or horses he has gone through, can take that away.

in sight. But you have just made it through another day. Good luck, my wonderful equine friends. I wish you a safe, healthy, and full recovery, a future, and a career. I wish you the best story ending, and your partner can dance again.

Your partner's owner will be okay too.

Chapter Eighteen
Rehabilitation Clinics

Therapy environments and rehabilitation clinics are available as an option as well. Your veterinarian may have some advice as to where they are located. We also must remember the Internet; the resources available there are vast. Remember to do your homework and investigate the options before you send your horse anyplace for this therapy, and make sure you are dealing with qualified professionals.

I highly recommend reading Dr. Hilary Clayton's book, *The Dynamic Horse*, for understanding the biomechanics of movement, as well as *Conditioning Sport Horses*. These books are invaluable for any person to gain knowledge of any aspect of equine movement. Also, Equine Lameness is a great book to have for a reference of multiple lameness issues.

The Internet will also offer a variety of links to visit and compare ideas and protocol procedures. It is a valuable tool of resources, and most of the information I discovered was fairly consistent.

About the Author

The original idea of the Plan Book started as a diary of experiences and notations. Rebecca had her horse, Hylynn Buddy, diagnosed with a digital flexor tendon injury in the year that the horse was ready to compete at the FEI levels. Only after a prior check ligament injury resulting from a trailer incident in the season of 2000. From the original injury in 2000 she knew what she was in for....again. She had to put all he dreams and goals on hold again, and realized their future was going to be limited simply because Buddy was not getting younger. She respected the fact that most FEI dressage horses need to be confirmed in the levels by a certain age. He lost the ability to "lift" his shoulders as a result of the last injury, challenging the movement and risking reinjury of the horse was not an option. As the days started to pass, she wrote down more organized ideas and started researching the factors involved in these types of injuries. This became her therapy and she focused on writing the research down and then focused her research in the form of a manual for other horseman to utilize if they found themselves faced with this issue. The failed stories she heard also motivated her, because "failure was not and option", One of her favorite quotes. "There must be a way to understand this issue and be successful at a level of soundness for the horse."

Rebecca graduated from the University of Massachusetts in 1989 with a BS, and a focus on Equine Studies and Art. She is also a USDF certified instructor. Her original plans included veterinary school but the quest of becoming an educated upper level trainer quickly got in the way. She became compelled to understand movement, theory and the bio-mechanics of the discipline of dressage. She was a working student with Sarah Geikie, Gerd Reuter, Tina Konyot and studies as often as she can with Felicitas Von Neuman Cosel.

Currently, she has a three year Dutch Stallion that she hopes to bring through the levels in the next few years. She lives in Florida during the winters with her husband Eric, and they manage a Water Park in New England during the summers. They have a cat, two good dogs and one bad basset hound, a donkey, Buddy now 19, and Elvis, Timmy and the queen Vixen.

She really hopes that this book helps give people some information and support.